THE LITTLE BOOK OF YOGA PRACTICES

*Daily Relaxation,
One Asana at a Time*

13-Digit ISBN: 978-1-60433-929-1
10-Digit ISBN: 1-60433-929-2

This book may be ordered by mail from the publisher. Please include $5.99 for postage and handling. Please support your local bookseller first!

Books published by Cider Mill Press Book Publishers are available at special discounts for bulk purchases in the United States by corporations, institutions, and other organizations. For more information, please contact the publisher.

Cider Mill Press Book Publishers
"Where Good Books Are Ready for Press"
PO Box 454
12 Spring Street
Kennebunkport, Maine 04046

Visit us online! www.cidermillpress.com

Typography: Agenda, Amatic, Avenir, Eplica, and Gotham
All photos used under official license from Shutterstock.com

Printed in China
1 2 3 4 5 6 7 8 9 0

The Little Book of Yoga Practices

Daily Relaxation, One Asana at a Time

RACHEL SCOTT

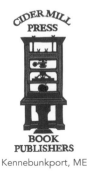

CIDER MILL PRESS

BOOK PUBLISHERS

Kennebunkport, ME

Contents

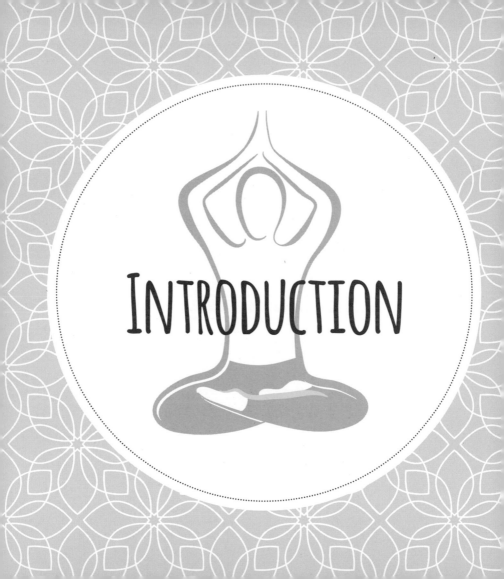

INTRODUCTION

The Power of the Micro Practice

When life is busy with kids, work, friends, and other obligations, you don't always have the luxury of taking two hours out of your day to attend a yoga class. But being busy doesn't mean that you can't practice yoga. In fact, the busier you are, the more important it becomes to carve out even just a few moments of "me time" to return to your center, clear your mind, and nourish your body with movement and breath. Your practice does not have to be long to be transformational; just 15 seconds of mindful breathing can be a powerful opportunity to regain perspective, awaken a sense of self, and restore your inner Zen.

By weaving micro practices into your everyday life, you will:

▶ Cultivate a consistent yoga routine that won't overwhelm your busy schedule
▶ Have the tools to reset your mood and energy with just a few breaths
▶ Feel empowered by the quality of your self-care
▶ Recognize that small acts can make a major difference in your physical and mental health

What You Need

You don't need anything fancy for these practices. An exercise may occasionally suggest a strap or a block, but you can easily substitute a towel and books for these props, respectively. You don't even need a yoga mat! Any non-slippery surface will work just fine. You can practice yoga on your living room rug or just using a towel.

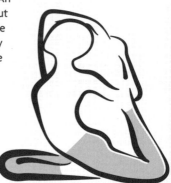

What is a Vinyasa?

Some of the practices include an invitation to "take a vinyasa." A vinyasa is a simple cycle of movements that includes the following postures:

▶ Begin in **Plank Pose** (see page 36).
▶ Exhale and lower halfway into **Four-Limbed Staff Pose** (see page 26) or all the way down to your mat.
▶ Inhale into a backbend like **Baby Cobra** (see page 15) or **Upward-Facing Dog** (see page 50).
▶ Exhale and lift up and back into **Downward-Facing Dog** (see page 20).

"Taking a vinyasa" helps create heat in the body, connects you to your breathing, and promotes the flow of energy. Vinyasa are always optional.

How to Use This Book

The first section of this book features detailed, step-by-step instructions to help guide you through a wide range of poses, while the second section offers over 30 micro practices to help nurture and strengthen your body. Whenever you need some inspiration, open this book to find a micro practice. You can select a specific practice that suits your situation and energy, or open to a random page for an impromptu experience. These practices are usually 5 to 15 minutes long, but feel free to shorten them by taking fewer breaths or skipping poses, or lengthen them by putting a couple of the micro practices together. You can also use this book as a reference for individual poses, or to create your own micro practice with targeted stretches for your body.

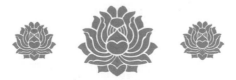

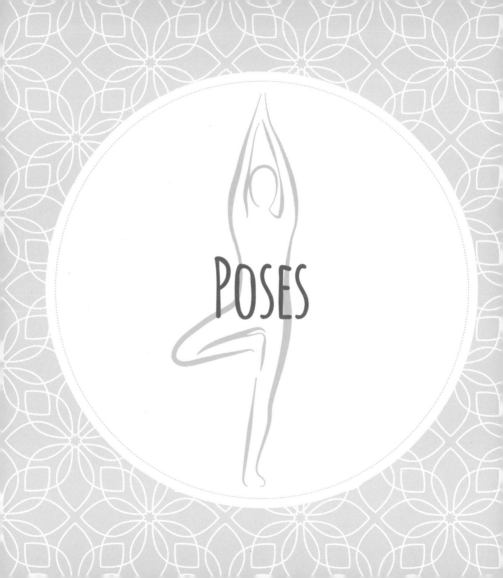

POSES

90/90 POSE

▶ From a seated position on your mat, place your right leg directly in front of you with your knee flat on the ground. Be sure to keep your leg at a right angle. Repeat this motion with your left leg, moving it behind you.

▶ Slowly bring your chest down toward your knee, keeping your shoulders squared and remembering to breathe. Keep your elbows close to your body unless they can reach your mat evenly, then rest them on your mat. Hold for 20 to 60 seconds, or lean further forward to intensify the stretch, completing 6 to 10 repetitions of 3 seconds each.

ABDOMINAL TWIST
(Jathara Parivartanasana)

▶ Lie on your back and bring your knees up to your chest. Breathe for 3 rounds to help relax your lower back. Then, place your arms out to the side at shoulder height with your palms facing upward. Exhale, then bring your knees over to the right and up toward your right elbow.

▶ Stretch your left arm away from your legs to deepen the twist. Press your left shoulder blade into your mat to help anchor the stretch. Exhale, then twist your chest further to the left. Round your lower back slightly to pull the stretch through your spine. Hold for 30 seconds, then bring your knees back to center. Repeat on the opposite side.

BABY COBRA
(Ardha Bhujangasana)

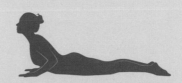

▶ Lie prone on your stomach and bring your hands under your shoulders, keeping your elbows tucked close to your body. Press the tops of your feet firmly down and lengthen your tailbone toward your heels.

▶ As you inhale, straighten your arms to lift your chest off the floor slightly, keeping your pelvis and legs connected to the ground. Draw your upper arms back slightly and bring your chest forward into a small backbend. Take 3 to 5 deep breaths. Slowly lower your upper body to your mat, and then press back into **Child's Pose** (see page 17) for several breaths.

BRIDGE POSE
(Setu Bandha Sarvangasana)

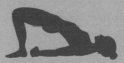

▶ Lie on your back, bend your legs, and place your feet flat on the floor so that your ankles are just below your knees. Allow your arms to rest along your side, palms facing down, and tuck your elbows in by your ribs.

▶ On an inhale, lift your hips up, keeping your thighs parallel. Press your tailbone downward. Lift your chest upward. Press the back of your head lightly down to keep your gaze looking up. To deepen your backbend, interlace your hands beneath your hips and press your upper arms into your mat to lift your chest. Take 5 deep breaths. Release your hands and slowly roll down through your spine to lie flat, continuing to breathe. Repeat 2 more times.

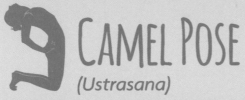

CAMEL POSE
(Ustrasana)

▶ Kneel with your knees and feet hip distance apart. Tuck your toes. Press your tailbone back and downward with your hands on your lower back. Lift through your torso and draw your lower belly in and up and your shoulders back and down.

▶ Hinging from your hips, bend your upper body back to a comfortable degree. If you feel secure, lean back and grasp your heels. Keeping your chin tucked to your chest, lift your chest up and bend your upper back, keeping your thighs parallel. Press your pelvis forward and bring the curve through your spine. Honor the position that feels supported in your lower back and breathe. To come out, bring your hands to your lower back and bring your upper body back to upright.

CAT/COW POSE
(Marjaryasana/Bitilasana)

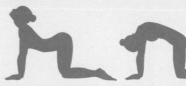

▶ Begin on your hands and knees. Place your palms under your shoulders and set your knees under your hips. As you inhale, drop your belly toward the earth, reach your chest forward through your arms, and tip your lower back up to the sky.

▶ As you exhale, press through your hands, look toward your belly, and round your spine upward. Continue arching and rounding your spine to find length through the front and back of your body. Link your breathing with the movement, feeling your body open on the inhale, and contract on the exhale.

Chair Pose
(Utkatasana)

▶ Begin in **Mountain Pose** (see page 34). Bring your toes together and your heels slightly apart. Press your legs together.

▶ On an exhale, bend your knees, sink your hips back, and tuck your tailbone down, keeping your weight centered on your heels. Reach your arms forward and up and relax your shoulders down your back. Engage your core. Sit deeper into the pose to strengthen your legs, back, and core. Remain for 5 slow breaths, then stand and release your arms to your sides. Take a breath and enjoy the strength of your body.

Child's Pose
(Balasana)

▶ Sit with your toes together and your knees a little wider than hip distance apart.

▶ Hinge forward from your hips to place your forehead on the earth or a block. Allow your arms to fall where feels comfortable. Check the position of your forehead against the floor and ensure that the skin of your forehead is wrinkling down toward the bridge of your nose rather than up. Let your face relax. Allow your head to get heavy and your belly to be soft and open. As you inhale, feel your breath move into your back ribs and lower back. As you exhale, allow any muscular tension to soften and let go. Remain in the pose for as long as feels nourishing. When you come out, take a few moments to stretch the backs of your knees by extending your legs back, or come into **Downward-Facing Dog** (see page 20).

COBRA POSE
(Bhujangasana)

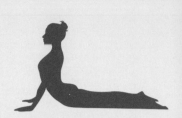

▶ Lie prone on your stomach and bring your hands under your shoulders, keeping your elbows tucked close to your body. Press the tops of your feet firmly down and lengthen your tailbone toward your heels.

▶ As you inhale, straighten your arms to lift your chest off the floor, keeping your pelvis and legs connected to the ground. Draw your upper arms back and bring your chest forward. Walk your hands closer in under your shoulders, stretching through your legs. Take 3 to 5 deep breaths. Slowly lower your upper body to your mat, and then press back into **Child's Pose** (see page 17) for several breaths.

CORPSE POSE
(Savasana)

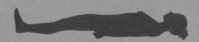

▶ Lie prone on your back with legs extended. Turn your palms up and lay them a few inches from your sides or on your chest and stomach. Let your body fully relax. Close your eyes. Take several long, smooth breaths and release the tension from your body. Let your breathing slow down. Remain in this pose for a least 5 minutes.

▶ To come out, draw your knees into your chest and roll onto your right side. Cradle your head on your right arm and take a few breaths. When you're ready to sit, use your top hand to press yourself slowly to a comfortable seat. Take a few slow breaths.

Cow Face Pose
(Gomukhasana)

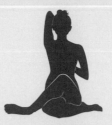

▶ Begin with your legs in front of you and your back straight, with your hands beside your hips. Bend your knees and bring your feet to rest on the floor. Bring your left foot under your right knee, then cross your right leg over your left, keeping your heels evenly apart from your hips. Rock slightly to balance your sitting position.

▶ Inhale and bring your right arm parallel to the floor. In one motion, rotate your arm so your palm faces the ceiling above your shoulder. Exhale and bring your right arm behind your torso, keeping your palm at the junction of your shoulder blades. Keep your right elbow parallel to your shoulder at all times. Repeat the circular stretching motion with your left arm, then bring your left arm behind your back and interlace your right and left hands. Lift your chest, hold for 1 minute, then reverse and repeat with your opposite leg on top.

DOWNWARD-FACING DOG
(Adho Mukha Svanasana)

▶ Begin on hands and knees. Turn your hands so your index fingers point forward and spread your fingers wide. Press into your fingers to take weight off of your wrists. Curl your toes under and lift your knees slightly.

▶ Keeping your knees bent, send your hips toward the sky. Press your index knuckles down and your forearms toward each other, then press your upper arms upward to relax your neck. Keeping your spine long, straighten your legs. Stretch from your hands through to your heels. Take 5 to 10 deep breaths. On your last exhale, slowly lower your knees and sit your hips back on your heels to come into **Child's Pose** (see page 17).

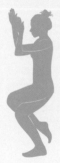

EAGLE POSE
(Garudasana)

▶ Stand in **Mountain Pose** (see page 34) with your hands on your hips. Bend your knees deeply to come into **Chair Pose** (see page 17). Press into your left foot and come onto the ball of your right foot. Turn your right knee inward about 45 degrees.

▶ From **Chair Pose**, lift your right leg as high as you can over your left thigh and squeeze the tops of your thighs together. Press your right shin into your left shin or wrap your right foot around your left calf. Lengthen your tailbone down, lifting your torso upward.

▶ Bring your arms wide, then wrap your arms. Hold on to your opposite shoulders or twine your forearms with palms together. Lift your elbows and press your forearms forward, opening your shoulder blades. Press into your standing foot, unwind your arms and legs, and release the pose. Repeat on the other side.

Easy Seat
(Sukhasana)

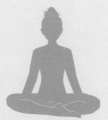

▶ Sit cross-legged, crossing at your shins. Switch legs so that your "non-traditional" shin is in front. Your shins should be placed far enough away that there is an open, triangular space between your hips and legs. Relax your legs fully. Rock slightly to find the center of your tailbone. Stretch your spine. Place your hands on your thighs and draw your arms back. Inhale and allow your ribs to expand. As you exhale, feel the subtle lifting of your pelvic floor. Soften your muscles, your face, and your eyes. Keeping the back of your neck long, tip your chin toward your chest until you feel a soft tension through the front of your throat, as if you were holding an orange beneath your chin. Your body is now ready to meditate.

Exalted Warrior Pose
(Viparita Virabhadrasana)

▶ Beginning in **Warrior 2** (see page 51), place your left palm on your left thigh. Turn your right palm upward and reach with your arm toward the ceiling. Deepen your backbend, being sure to support the stretch in your lower back. Tilt your chin upward to help relax your neck, being sure to push your shoulders back and down and keep your tailbone angled down.

▶ Maintaining your backbend, lean on your right knee, keeping your knee in line with your ankle. Hold for 5 to 10 breaths, then come out of the backbend and come up into **Mountain Pose** (see page 34).

Extended Cat Pose
(Utthita Marjaryasana)

▶ Starting in the center of your mat, come into **Tabletop Pose** (see page 47), keeping your hips aligned with your knees and your shoulders in line with your wrists. Keeping your neck relaxed downward, lean onto your left hand and extend your right arm forward, pointing your thumb toward the ceiling.

▶ Lift your stomach upward into a slight backbend and stretch your right leg behind you, with your toes resting on the ground. Once you feel comfortably balanced, lift your right toes off of the ground and stretch your leg out behind you. Be sure to keep your hips level and your shoulder blades stretched along your spine. Hold for 3 to 5 breaths, return to **Tabletop Pose**, and repeat on the opposite side.

Extended Child's Pose
(Utthita Balasana)

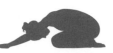

▶ Begin in **Child's Pose** (see page 17). Rest your weight on your heels and extend your arms up and over your shoulders, coming to rest with them in a triangle shape in front of you. Round your spine and slowly move downward until your forehead rests firmly on the ground and your fingers are either spread wide or on top of each other. Allow your body to fully relax into your mat, keeping your hips in contact with your heels. Hold for as long as feels nourishing. When you come out, take a few moments to stretch the backs of your knees by extending your legs back, or move into **Downward-Facing Dog** (see page 20).

Extended Hand-to-Foot Pose
(Utthita Hasta Padangusthasana)

▶ Begin in **Mountain Pose** (see page 34). Then, bring your left knee up and toward your stomach. Move your left arm along the inside of your left thigh, then cross it over your left ankle and hold on to the outside of your foot. If this position is too tight on your hamstrings, you can use a strap around your foot.

▶ Press into your right leg and bring your left thigh inward. Inhale and extend your left leg outward. Straighten your knee as far as possible. You can stay here, or extend your leg out to the side if you feel balanced. Hold for 30 seconds, then bring your leg back to center on an inhale and to the floor on an exhale. Repeat on the opposite side, then return to **Mountain Pose**.

Eye of the Needle Pose

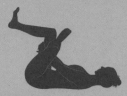

(Sucirandhrasana)

▶ Begin in **Hero's Pose** (see page 30), then recline onto your back. Cross your right ankle over your left knee and draw your left knee into your chest, keeping the back of your shin against your thigh. Breathe into the tightness of your outer hip and allow your right hip to settle toward your body. Close your eyes and let your head rest onto the floor. Take 10 deep breaths, then slowly change sides.

Finger Stand Cobra

(Bhujangasana, Variation)

▶ Begin on your stomach with your legs extended behind you and your feet flat on your mat, keeping your legs slightly apart and in line with your hips. Bring your hands out to either side of your chest, just past the edge of your mat. Bend your elbows so they point upward, then raise the palms of your hands until you are resting on the tips of your fingers in a claw-like position.

▶ Press your feet, legs, hips, and fingertips into your mat to support your body, then lift your head and chest upward. Pull your stomach inward and press your tailbone downward to support your body, arching your back as you do so. Lift your chest and head upward, dropping your shoulders back and outward as you do so to deepen your stretch. Straighten your arms almost all the way, keeping your elbows slightly bent. Hold for 3 to 6 breaths, then lower your torso back to the floor, focusing on your breathing.

Forearm Plank

(Phalakasana, Forearm Variation)

▶ Come to your hands and knees with your hands under your shoulders and your knees under your hips. Come down onto your forearms and step one foot back at a time. Lift your hips to the level of your shoulders, and then lengthen your tailbone back to your heels to engage your core and support your lower back.

▶ Lift your front ribs in as you draw your shoulder blades closer together and expand your chest. Press back through your heels as you reach your chest forward. After 30 seconds to 1 minute, lower your knees softly to your mat, press back into **Child's Pose** (see page 17), and take a few deep breaths.

Forward Fold

(Uttanasana)

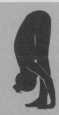

▶ Stand with your feet hip distance apart and parallel. Inhale, roll your shoulders back, and lift your chest to lengthen your spine.

▶ As you exhale, bend your knees and hinge forward from your hips. If possible, bring your chest onto your thighs so that your upper body is supported by your legs. Fold forward as deeply as you can with a straight spine, allow your back to round, and release your head toward the earth. Take a few deep breaths, feeling the backs of your legs open and releasing any tension through your neck and jaw. Let your upper body hang heavy. To come out, relax your knees, bring your hands to your hips, and lift your shoulders. Press through your feet and slowly rise to stand.

FOUR-LIMBED STAFF POSE
(Chaturanga Dandasana)

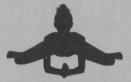

▶ Begin in **Plank Pose** (see page 36). Push your shoulder blades back and down and angle your tailbone toward the front of your hips. Exhale, then lower yourself down until your body and legs are a few inches above the floor and parallel to your mat. Focus on keeping your tailbone level with the rest of your body, tensing your stomach to help lift your hips.

▶ Be sure to keep your shoulders stretched and your elbows close to your body. Pressing into your index fingers, lift the front of your chest upward and look forward. Hold for 10 to 30 seconds. Exhale, then either come to lay on your mat or shift back into **Downward-Facing Dog** (see page 20).

FROG POSE
(Mandukasana)

▶ Begin facing the long edge of your mat, then come into **Tabletop Pose** (see page 47). Walk your knees out to either side so they are wider than your hips. You should feel a deep stretch through the insides of your hips. If you feel any discomfort, bring your knees closer together.

▶ Turn your feet to either side, so they are perpendicular to the long edge of your mat. Move your heels directly behind your knees, and lean your arms and chest forward to come to rest on your forearms. If necessary, add a block under your forearms or hips to help support your body. Focus on stretching your head forward and angling your tailbone back. Your hips should stay above your knees to prevent undue strain. Lift your stomach in and back and hold this pose for up to 2 minutes. Move your knees back toward the center of your mat and come into **Child's Pose** (see page 17).

GODDESS POSE
(Utkata Konasana)

▶ Begin in **Mountain Pose** (see page 34). Then, turn toward the long side of your mat and bring your feet approximately 3 feet apart. Turn your heels in and your toes out, so your feet are at a 45-degree angle. Exhale, bend your knees, and bring your thighs parallel to your mat with your hips over your knees. Be sure your knees stay above your heels in order to feel the full effect of the stretch.

▶ Bring your arms out and to the side at shoulder height, then bend your elbows to right angles with your palms facing outward. Spread your fingers and bring your shoulder blades back and out. Tense your core and bring your lower ribs back and up. Center your tailbone over your hips, keeping your shoulders in line with your hips. Stretch through your heels and hold the pose for 5 breaths. To come out, stand upright, lower your arms, and return to **Mountain Pose**.

Half Sun Salutation

(Ardha Surya Namaskar)

▶ Begin in **Mountain Pose** (see page 34). Make sure your back is fully stretched and relax your shoulders. Then, inhale and reach your arms outward and upward for **Upward Salute** (see page 49). Bring your palms together above your head or allow them to stay shoulder distance apart. Look upward to relax your neck.

▶ Exhale and bend your knees slightly into **Forward Fold** (see page 25). Allow your body to relax into the fold. Be sure to center on your feet, as leaning too far back can put undue strain on your hips.

▶ Inhale and come up into **Halfway Lift** (see facing page). Be sure to keep your spine flat by moving your hands to the most comfortable position on your legs.

▶ Exhale back into **Forward Fold**. If desired, rest here for 2 to 3 breaths to help fully release your spine.

▶ Inhale and rise up, reaching your arms back up for **Upward Salute** with your shoulders even and spread outward.

▶ Exhale and bring your hands to your sides to return to **Mountain Pose**. Repeat these poses 4 times, focusing on the connection of your movement with your breathing.

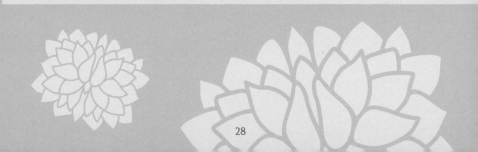

Halfway Lift
(Ardha Uttanasana)

▶ Begin in **Forward Fold** (see page 25). Place your hands on either your shins or the floor in front of your feet. Inhale, straighten your arms, and unfold your torso outward as far as you can, creating a space between your pelvis and navel.

▶ Pushing down with your hands, lift your sternum up and forward. Bend your knees as you arch your back, allowing the stretch to move through your shoulders and over the curve of your back down to your waist. Keeping your eyes forward and your neck long, hold the position for a few breaths. Exhale and return to **Forward Fold**.

Happy Baby
(Ananda Balasana)

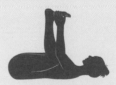

▶ Lying on your back, exhale and bend your knees to your stomach. Inhale, grabbing the outside of your feet and bringing them upward. If you have difficulty fully stretching your legs, you can use a strap to hold your feet. Open your knees slightly wider than your hips, keeping your shins perpendicular to the floor. Push your heels into your hands, pressing down with your hands to deepen the stretch. Hold for 5 breaths, then relax back to a lying position.

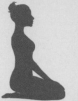

HERO'S POSE
(Virasana)

▶ Stack one or two blocks on top of each other. Sit on the blocks so that your ankles hug the outside of the blocks and your thighs are close and parallel to each other. Adjust your sitting height as needed for comfort. Rock slightly to find the center of your tailbone. Place your hands on your upper thighs, with palms facing up or down. Draw your arms back to widen your collarbones. Inhale and feel your lungs and ribs expand. As you exhale, feel the subtle lifting of your pelvic floor. Soften your muscles, your face, and your eyes. Keeping the back of your neck long, tip your chin toward your chest until you feel a soft tension through the front of your throat, as if you were holding an orange beneath your chin.

HIGH-CRESCENT LUNGE

▶ Begin in **Downward-Facing Dog** (see page 20) and raise your right leg toward the sky.
▶ Step your right foot to your right thumb, keeping your feet hip distance apart. Place your hand on your front thigh and lift your torso up to come into a high lunge. Lengthen your tailbone downward and straighten your back leg, keeping your left heel lifted. Reach your arms up by your ears into a wide Y shape. Lift your chest forward and up for a gentle backbend. Hold for 5 deep breaths and feel your inner body expand and open. On your final exhale, slowly bring your hands to the floor, step into **Downward-Facing Dog**, and take a few breaths before repeating on the other side.

INTERRUPTED BREATHING EXERCISE
(Viloma Pranayama)

▶ Begin in **Easy Seat** (see page 21) or **Hero's Pose** (see page 30). Place one hand on your belly and one hand on your lower ribs. Take a full breath in and out to prepare. Take a modest inhale into your belly. Pause. Take a modest inhale into your lower ribs. Pause. Take a final inhale into your upper chest. Pause. Exhale all the way out. Repeat this for 6 rounds, then return to your natural breathing.

KNEES-TO-CHEST POSE
(Apanasana)

▶ Lying prone on your back, bend your right knee toward your chest, keeping your left leg straight. Place your hands under your knee, lacing your fingers. Flex your left foot toward you, stretching your hip. Hug your knee closer toward your armpit, relaxing your neck and shoulders. Pull your shoulder blades outward, stretching your upper back. Breathe deeply, lengthening your spine and drawing your tailbone downward. Release your hands, straighten your leg, and repeat on the other side.

LEGS-UP-THE-WALL POSE
(Viparita Karani)

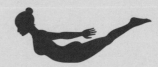

▶ Sit about a foot away from the wall. Lie on your side and swing your legs up the wall. For tighter hamstrings, position your pelvis further from the wall. Take a position where your legs can comfortably relax. Keep your chin level with the floor, adding a book behind your head if needed. Allow your back to completely relax into the floor, and let your legs relax and settle into the wall. Remain for about 5 minutes. To come out, bend your knees first into your chest, then slowly roll to one side. Take your time to come up, and sit quietly for a few moments.

LOCUST POSE
(Salabhasana)

▶ Lie on your stomach with your arms at your sides, palms facing down. Press the tops of your feet firmly down, keeping your legs parallel. Lengthen your tailbone toward your heels. Roll your shoulders down your back and exhale.

▶ On an inhale, lift the whole length of your body, keeping your gaze down. Stretch your hands back toward your heels. Reach back through your toes, keeping your legs parallel. Focus on the length of the stretch instead of height. Stay for 3 breaths, breathing into your upper chest. On your last exhale, lower your body and release your hands. Turn your head to one side and completely let go. Repeat. After 3 rounds, take a few breaths and return to **Child's Pose** (see page 17).

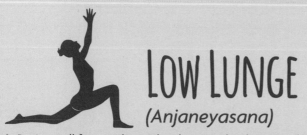

Low Lunge
(Anjaneyasana)

▶ Begin on all fours with your hands just wider than your shoulders and your knees just behind your hips. Place your right foot by your right thumb. Bring your hands to your right thigh to lift your torso upward. Square your hips with your tailbone pointing down. Settle your hips forward and down to stretch the front of your left thigh. Be sure to keep your knee over your right heel.

▶ Draw your front ribs in and reach your arms forward and up in a wide V. Press your thighs together for stability. Draw your chest out into a mini backbend. Stretch through the length of your torso and out through your fingertips. Take 3 deep breaths. You can choose to keep your left knee down or lifted. As you exhale, bring your hands to your front thigh and then your mat. Step your right foot back, take a few breaths in **Child's Pose** (see page 17), and repeat on the other side.

Mountain Pose
(Tadasana)

▶ Stand with your feet either hip distance apart or together and parallel to each other. Lift your toes and stretch your inner and outer arches. Keeping your arches lightly stretched, relax your toes and press your feet downward. Engage the top of your thighs, with your tailbone pointing down and pelvis even. Draw your lower belly slightly in and up, then inhale and lengthen your waist. Roll your shoulders back and down and stretch your fingertips downward. Relax your front ribs in and down and draw your shoulder blades slightly together. Stretch your neck so your chin is level with the floor. Relax your eyes and take 5 to 10 deep breaths, becoming aware of the strength of your body.

Nesting Eagle Pose

(Garudasana, Variation)

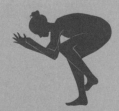

▶ Begin in **Eagle Pose** (see page 20). Swing your left arm under your right and either hold on to opposite shoulders or twine your forearms and press your palms together. Take 2 deep breaths, then hinge from your hips to come forward with your elbows in front of your knees. Hold this pose for 5 to 10 breaths. To come out, lift your torso upward, untwine your arms, and untwist your legs, coming out into **Mountain Pose** (see above).

One-Legged Chair Pose

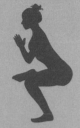

(Eka Pada Utkatasana)

▶ Begin in **Chair Pose** (see page 17). Hold for 4 breaths, making sure to keep your thighs down low and your body weight shifted to your heels. Bring your palms together in front of your chest. Keeping your weight on your left foot, bring your right foot up and cross your right ankle over your left knee. Your legs should form a triangle opening with your hips. Hold this pose for 3 to 5 breaths.

▶ To deepen the stretch, lean your chest forward until your hands rest on your right calf. Depending on your personal balance, you can continue to lean forward until your fingers touch the floor, or you can release your right leg to the floor to return to **Chair Pose** before coming out of the pose.

Pelvic Clock

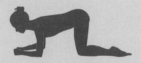

▶ Begin by bringing your knees completely to one side. Roll over onto that side and come onto all fours with your knees under your hips. Place your elbows under your shoulders, interlace your hands, and move your hips in a big, lazy circle to open your lower back and your shoulders. Move in one direction for about 5 rounds, then change directions. To come out, move up onto all fours and either stand up or lean forward into **Downward-Facing Dog** (see page 20).

PIGEON POSE

(Eka Pada Kapotasana)

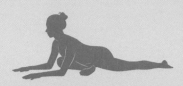

▶ Beginning on hands and knees, bring your right knee to rest on the floor behind your right hand. Angle your right foot toward the left side of your mat, stretching your hip and not your knee. Flex your foot to stabilize the pose.

▶ Slowly extend your left leg straight back until it rests on the floor. Lift your pelvis, squaring it to your mat. If your right hip raises, rest on a blanket or block. Exhale and slowly walk your hands forward. Bring your torso to rest on the floor, or rest on your elbows. Hold for 5 breaths. Walk your hands back to rest slightly wider than shoulder width. Lift your collarbones and inhale to return upright. Hold for 5 breaths, then move into **Child's Pose** (see page 17).

PLANK POSE

(Kumbhakasana)

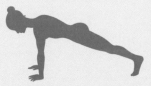

▶ Come onto your hands and knees with hands under your shoulders and knees under your hips. Press into your hands and step one foot back at a time. Lift your hips to the level of your shoulders, and then lengthen your tailbone back to your heels to engage your core and support your lower back.

▶ Lift your front ribs in as you draw your shoulder blades closer together and expand your chest. Press back through your heels as you reach your chest forward. After 30 seconds to 1 minute, lower your knees softly to your mat, press back into **Child's Pose** (see page 17), and take a few deep breaths.

Prone Corpse Pose

(Supta Savasana)

▶ Begin on your stomach with your hands at your sides and legs out behind you. Bend your right knee and bring it in line with your right hip. Move your arms above your head and turn your face to the right. Relax completely. Take at least 5 breaths, then change sides. If needed, you can add a blanket or block under your hips or head to make this pose more comfortable.

Pyramid Pose

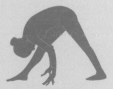

(Parsvottanasana)

▶ Begin in **Mountain Pose** (see page 34) and breathe deeply. On an exhale, spread your feet about 4 feet apart. Raise your arms upward, pushing your shoulder blades back and down to extend the stretch. Position both feet to point forward. Exhale and turn your torso toward your front foot. Level your hips and arch your upper torso slightly to find your balance.

▶ On an exhale, hinge your torso toward the floor, bending at your hips. Bring your fingertips to the floor or on blocks. Stretch through your front thigh and relax your head toward the floor. Keeping your hips level, bring your torso closer to your thigh. Hold for 15 to 30 seconds, then rise on the inhale. Repeat on the other side.

Reclined Cow Face Pose
(Supta Gomukhasana)

▶ Lie on your back and cross your right knee over the left. Inhale and grasp your ankles. Exhale and draw your feet toward the floor on either side of your waist. If you cannot fully bring your ankles to the floor, you can rest them on blocks for added support. Hold for 10 to 15 breaths.

▶ Unwind, come back to a neutral pose on your back, then switch to the opposite side.

Reclined Hand-to-Foot Pose
(Supta Padangusthasana)

This pose works best with a strap or towel, and can be done with a folded blanket for support.

▶ Lie on your back with your legs extended. Rest your head on the floor or a folded blanket, keeping your spine even. Exhale, then bend your left knee and bring your left thigh to your chest. Hug your thigh to your stomach, pressing down through your right thigh and heel to deepen the stretch.

▶ Place the strap around the arch of your left foot, holding the ends of the strap in both hands. Inhale, straighten your knee, and press your left heel upward. Adjust your hands on the strap until your elbows are straight. Widen your shoulder blades outward, then press them into your mat, keeping your hands as high on the strap as you can. Be sure to keep your chest flattened toward your mat.

▶ To deepen your stretch, extend your leg from the heel upward until you feel a strong stretch through your body. If possible, bring your foot closer to your head to fully release your hamstrings. Hold this pose for 1 to 3 minutes, then repeat on the opposite side.

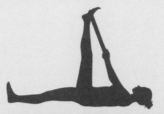

RECLINED MOUNTAIN POSE
(Supta Tadasana)

This pose requires blankets or blocks to support the body.

▶ Arrange 2 blocks or blankets with one at the top of your mat and one near the bottom with room for your feet. Sit in the center of your mat facing the short end. Be sure to give yourself enough support under your knees to take some of the stress of this pose off of your lower back.

▶ Recline back with your head on the top block or blanket and your knees bent over the lower prop. Bring your hands to rest on either side and allow a gentle backbend to come into your lower back. If desired, support your lower back with an additional blanket. Hold this pose for 5 to 10 minutes, then slowly come up to a sitting position or remove the props and come into **Corpse Pose** (see page 18).

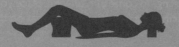

REVOLVED CHAIR POSE
(Parivrtta Utkatasana)

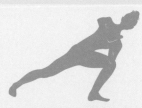

▶ Begin in **Chair Pose** (see page 17). Balance back on your heels and bring your hands together in front of you with your palms facing each other. Inhale and stretch through your spine. Then, exhale and bend forward, twisting to the right side and looping your left elbow outside of your right thigh to provide additional balance.

▶ Press your palms firmly together to help stretch your shoulder blades. Keeping your knees closely together, lower your hips down slightly, being sure to maintain your balance throughout the pose. Hold for 3 to 5 breaths, then bend forward into **Forward Fold** (see page 25). Return to **Chair Pose** and repeat on the opposite side.

REVOLVED LUNGE
(Parivrtta Anjaneyasana)

▶ Begin in **Low Lunge** (see page 33) with your right leg forward. Press your palms together at the center of your chest. Lift your left knee, bring your heel back, and press upward with your head, lengthening your spine.

▶ On an exhale, twist your torso toward your right leg. Keeping your palms together, rest your left triceps on your right thigh. Lengthen your spine as you inhale and twist deeper as you exhale. Hold this pose for 1 minute or reach one hand downward and the other toward the ceiling. To come out, unwind, place your palms on your mat, and step into **Downward-Facing Dog** (see page 20). Repeat on the opposite side.

Revolved Side Angle Pose

(Parivrtta Parsvakonasana)

▶ Begin in **Warrior I** (see page 50) with your left foot forward and your right foot back. Place your hands on your hips.

▶ Exhale, twist left, and bring your torso down. Place your right arm along the outside of your left knee with your hand on the floor or a block. Raise your left arm alongside your head and stretch, softening your stomach. Hold for 30 seconds to 1 minute, inhale, and return upright. Exhale to undo the twist. Repeat on the opposite side, then come into **Mountain Pose** (see page 34).

Saddle Pose

(Supta Virasana)

▶ Begin in **Hero Pose** (see page 30).

▶ With a back support prepared if needed, exhale and lower your lower back, leaning on your hands, then your forearms, and finally your elbows to support you. Then, place your hands behind your pelvis and release your lower back and upper thigh muscles. Allow yourself to fully recline onto the floor or the back support. If your ribs point upward, use your hands to press down on your ribs and lift your pelvis toward your navel, or adjust your support. If needed, you can add a blanket under your knees to lessen the strain on your hips. Keep your knees even with your hips to prevent strain as well. Hold for 30 seconds to 1 minute. To come out, press into your forearms and raise using the pressure on your hands, leading with your sternum until you return to **Hero's Pose**.

SIDE ANGLE POSE
(Parsvakonasana)

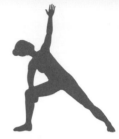

▶ Stand facing the long side of your mat. Lift your arms out to shoulder height and step so that your ankles are under your wrists. Turn your right leg so your right toes point to the short end of your mat. Align your right heel with the arch of your left foot and tilt in your left toes. Bend your right knee until it is over your ankle.

▶ Shift your hips back and place your right forearm on your right thigh. Press your knee toward your front foot and bring your tailbone down and back. Press your right forearm down and draw your right shoulder back. Sweep your left arm over your ear and turn your chest slightly upward. Stretch through the tips of your fingers. Hold for 5 breaths. To come out, press into your front heel and inhale to lift your torso up, straightening your legs. Repeat on the left side.

SKULL-SHINING BREATH
(Kapalabhati)

▶ To begin, sit either on the floor, on a block, or on the edge of a chair. Lift tall through your spine and reach your arms overhead in a wide V position. Take a deep inhale, then exhale fully. Inhale halfway, then begin a series of short, sharp exhales through your nose at a rate of about 1 to 2 per second. Allow your inhales to drop in naturally and keep your chest lifted and open. Exhale 25 times. Take a few natural breaths in and out to conclude the pose.

Sphinx Pose
(Salamba Bhujangasana)

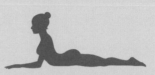

▶ Begin lying prone. Press the tops of your feet firmly down and lengthen your tailbone toward your heels to engage your core.

▶ On an inhale, prop yourself up on your forearms with your elbows under your shoulders. If you feel any discomfort, walk your elbows further forward. Roll your shoulders back and down, pull your forearms toward you, and push your chest forward. Pull your bottom ribs in slightly to widen your back, and exhale. Take 3 to 5 deep breaths. Slowly lower your upper body to the earth, and then press back into **Child's Pose** (see page 17) for several breaths.

Standing Backbend
(Anuvittasana)

▶ Begin in **Mountain Pose** (see page 34) with feet hip distance apart. Pull up through your legs, stretching through them until your knees feel higher. Keep your tailbone angled downward while drawing your stomach up and back and your chest forward. Allow your shoulders to relax.

▶ Place your palms on the center of your lower back, with your fingers pointing downward. Draw your elbows back and toward each other. Inhale and focus in on your core. Exhale and bend your spine back, being sure not to exceed what feels comfortable. Adjust your neck so it is in line with your spine, or tilt backward and allow to relax. Hold for 3 to 5 breaths, focusing on relaxing your chest and deepening your backbend. To come out, inhale and return to **Mountain Pose** slowly, using your palms to help bring your spine to an upright position.

STANDING SIDE BEND
(Parsva Urdhva Hastasana)

▶ Begin in **Mountain Pose** (see page 34). Inhale and sweep your arms upward, reaching to press your palms together. If your shoulders are too tight, stop when your arms are parallel to your shoulders. Stretch through your arms and neck, tilting your head upward. Bring your ribs down and in, reaching your tailbone downward. Lift your chest upward to stretch your belly and hold for 5 breaths.

▶ Tilt your pose, starting at your hips and curving your side. Reach your arms to the same side, curving your whole torso. Breathe for 5 breaths, then repeat on the other side.

▶ Come back to center, bring your arms out to the side, and tilt your torso down into **Forward Fold** (see page 25).

STANDING SPLIT
(Urdhva Prasarita Eka Padasana)

▶ Begin in **High-Crescent Lunge** (see page 30) with your right leg forward. Lean forward and bring your torso to rest on your right thigh. Place your hands on the floor on either side of your right foot or a block.

▶ Walk your hands ahead of your right foot, shifting your weight to your right foot. Inhale and straighten your right leg, lifting your left leg upward. To maintain your balance, keep your hips and knees squared toward the front of your mat. Focus on pulling the stretch evenly through your body and hold for 30 seconds to 1 minute. On the exhale, lower your leg and repeat on the other side.

Sun Salutation A
(Surya Namaskar A)

▶ Stand in **Mountain Pose** (see page 34) with your feet hip distance apart and parallel.

▶ As you inhale, reach your arms up to the sky into **Upward Salute** (see page 49).

▶ As you exhale, **Forward Fold** (see page 25) and bring your fingers to the earth.

▶ As you inhale, bring your fingertips to your shins, and lift halfway up into a mini backbend.

▶ As you exhale, place your palms to the earth shoulder distance apart and step back into **Plank Pose** (see page 36).

▶ As you continue to exhale, slowly lower halfway or fully down to the earth into **Four-Limbed Staff Pose** (see page 26).

▶ As you inhale, reach your chest forward and up into **Cobra Pose** (see page 18) or **Upward-Facing Dog** (see page 50).

▶ As you exhale, engage your core and reach your hips up and back to come into **Downward-Facing Dog** (see page 20). Take 5 deep breaths.

▶ After 5 exhales, step or walk your feet to the front of your mat. Inhale, bring your fingertips to your shins, and lift halfway up into a mini backbend.

▶ Exhale into a **Forward Fold** with your fingertips on the earth.

▶ Inhale, press through your feet, and reach your arms up into the sky for **Upward Salute**.

▶ Exhale and bring your hands to your sides to come back into **Mountain Pose**. Repeat up to 5 times, and feel your whole body expand in this moving meditation.

Sun Salutation B
(Surya Namaskar B)

▶ Begin in **Mountain Pose** (see page 34). Bend your knees, then inhale and reach your arms up to the sky for **Chair Pose** (see page 17).

▶ Exhale into **Forward Fold** (see page 25). On the inhale, come into **Halfway Lift** (see page 29).

▶ Exhale, step back into **Plank Pose** (see page 36), and lower down into **Four-Limbed Staff Pose** (see page 26).

▶ Inhale into a backbend, then exhale to **Downward-Facing Dog** (see page 20).

▶ Step your right foot to your right thumb, lower your back knee, if desired, and reach your arms up into **High-Crescent Lunge** (see page 30).

▶ As you exhale, lower your hands to the earth and step back into a vinyasa or into **Downward-Facing Dog** for 5 deep breaths.

▶ Step your left foot to your left thumb and inhale to rise up into **High-Crescent Lunge** on the other side, and repeat the sequence.

▶ At the end of your last exhale in **Downward-Facing Dog**, walk, step, or jump your feet forward.

▶ Inhale into **Halfway Lift**, then exhale into **Forward Fold**.

▶ Inhale and bend your knees into **Chair Pose**.

▶ Exhale into **Mountain Pose**. Repeat the sequence, including the side switch, two more times, focusing on linking your breathing with your movement.

Supported Child's Pose with Twist

(Parivrtta Balasana)

This pose requires blankets or other props.

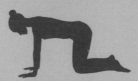

▶ Begin in **Child's Pose** (see page 17) with your knees wider than your hips and two or more blankets stacked at the short end of your mat. Point your toes backward, then slide the blankets between your thighs to support your chest and hips.

▶ Lean back into your heels. Lift up partway, then thread your right arm underneath your left to wrap around the blanket. You can rest your head on a block or book, if desired. Take 5 breaths, then change sides.

Tabletop Pose

(Bharmanasana)

▶ Begin on your hands and knees with your knees hip distance apart and your palms directly under your shoulders. Look down at your hands and flatten your back, stretching through your spine and focusing on keeping your body stable. Press into your palms to relax your shoulders down and back. Press your tailbone back to stretch your spine. Hold the pose for 1 to 3 breaths, then come down into **Child's Pose** (see page 17) or step back into **Downward-Facing Dog** (see page 20).

Thread the Needle Pose

(Parsva Balasana)

▶ Begin in **Tabletop Pose** (see page 47), being sure your shoulders are above your wrists and your hips are above your knees. Inhale, then reach your right arm out and upward. Exhale and loop your right arm underneath your left arm. Lower your right shoulder and ear to your mat, stretching your right arm through the space created by your left arm to deepen the stretch.

▶ Be sure to balance your weight through your knees and feet, keeping your feet securely on your mat. Hold for 5 to 10 breaths, return to **Tabletop Pose**, and repeat on the opposite side.

Three-Legged Downward-Facing Dog

(Eka Pada Adho Mukha Svanasana)

▶ Begin in **Downward-Facing Dog** (see page 20).

▶ Bring your left foot up and back, straightening your knee. Press back to feel the stretch, but do not over extend your hip. Keep your weight focused on your palms to help maintain your balance. Draw your tailbone back and your head forward toward the floor, bringing the stretch from your heel to your head. Hold for 5 to 10 breaths, then return to **Downward-Facing Dog** and repeat on the other side.

TREE POSE
(Vrksasana)

▶ Start near a wall or chair for added support. Stand in **Mountain Pose** (see page 34) and place your hands on your hips. Keeping your hands on your hips, press your left foot down and come onto the ball of your right foot. Turn your right knee out about 45 degrees. Place the sole of your right foot onto your left ankle, shin, or thigh above your knee.

▶ Press your foot into your standing leg. Lift from your torso to the crown of your head. Connect your palms together in front of your heart. If you feel steady, reach your arms overhead to enjoy a full stretch through the length of your body. To come out, bring your hands back together in front of your heart, turn your right knee forward, and then step your foot down. Repeat on the other side.

UPWARD SALUTE
(Urdhva Hastasana)

▶ Stand in **Mountain Pose** (see page 34) with your feet hip distance apart.

▶ Lift your arms up into a wide V above your head and stretch toward the sky through your fingertips, lengthening through the sides of your body. Relax the muscles at the base of your neck, draw your upper arms back by your ears, and open your chest. Breathe deeply. Stay in this pose for 2 minutes, continuing to stretch your whole body. After 2 minutes, relax your arms and take a few deep breaths.

UPWARD-FACING DOG
(Urdhva Mukha Svanasana)

▶ Lie prone on your stomach and bring your hands under your shoulders. Press the tops of your feet down to engage your legs. Lengthen your tailbone toward your heels, then lift your shoulders and roll them back.

▶ Press into your hands and lift your chest, then straighten your arms and lift your legs and pelvis off the floor. Press through the tops of your feet, relax your elbows, and press your chest forward, relaxing your upper arms. Lengthen the back of your neck. Take 3 breaths into your upper chest. To come up, draw your core in and up and lift your pelvis up and back to come into **Downward-Facing Dog** (see page 20). Lower your knees and come into **Child's Pose** (see page 17).

WARRIOR 1
(Virabhadrasana 1)

▶ Begin in **Mountain Pose** (see page 34) at the front of your mat.

▶ Step your left foot about 3 feet behind you. Position your left foot so it is at a 45-degree angle and your right foot points forward. Square your shoulders and hips toward the front of your mat. Bend your right leg until it reaches a right angle, aligning knee over ankle. Raise your arms upward and glide your shoulder blades down your back. Press your chest upward toward your raised arms. Arch your back slightly to find your balance. To come out, bring your arms to your sides as you step your left foot forward, breathing deeply into your opened chest. Repeat on the left side.

WARRIOR 2
(Virabhadrasana 2)

► Stand in the center of your mat and face the long side.

► Step your right foot forward and left foot back, about 4 feet apart. Keeping your hips and shoulders facing the long edge of your mat, bend your right knee so it is above your ankle. Align your right heel with the arch of your left foot, tilting your left toes inward so the outer edge of your left foot is parallel with the back of your mat. Lift from your pelvis and stretch through your torso. Ease your shoulders down and away from your ears, stretch your arms wide at shoulder height, and turn your head to look over your right fingertips. Take 5 slow breaths. Slowly straighten your right leg and turn your right thigh until parallel with your left. Lower your hands to your hips, inhale, and repeat on the left side.

WARRIOR 3
(Virabhadrasana 3)

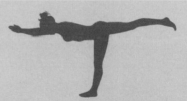

► Stand facing the wall and place your fingertips on the wall at hip height. Make sure your hands are shoulder distance apart. Press your palms into the wall and step your feet back until your ankles are directly under your hips. Place your feet together and press your legs inward, bending your knees. Reach your hips back into the center of the room and stretch your spine fully, keeping your head directly between your arms.

► Keep your right leg straight and lift your left leg until level with your back, forming a T shape. Keep your hips square, stretching your inner left thigh upward and pushing your outer right hip back. Stretch fully through the length of your body and breathe. Slowly lower your left foot down to come back into an L shape. Repeat on the other side.

WIDE-LEGGED FORWARD FOLD

(Prasarita Padottanasana 1)

▶ Begin in **Mountain Pose** (see page 34). Exhale, place your hands on your hips, and spread your feet about 4 feet apart parallel to each other. With a straight torso, bend at the hips. Place your fingertips on the floor under your shoulders, keeping your torso parallel to the ground. Look toward the floor, keeping your neck straight.

▶ On an exhale, bend your elbows and torso to move into a full forward bend, walking your torso back and down using your hands. Rest your hands on the ground where comfortable. Let your head and neck relax down. Hold for 30 seconds to 1 minute. To come out, bring your hands under your shoulders, press your torso up, and, with hands on hips, step your feet back to return to **Mountain Pose**.

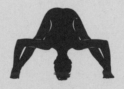

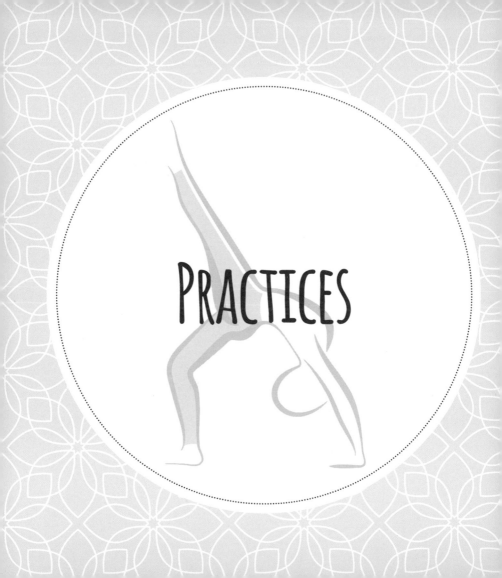

PRACTICES

Morning Awakenings

Sweet Morning Flow

▶ Come into **Extended Child's Pose** (see page 23) by bringing your hips back to your heels. Rest your forehead on your hands, a book, a block, or the floor. Gently roll your forehead side to side on the block to release any tension in your forehead.

▶ Keeping your left hip anchored back and down, walk your hands over to the right side of your mat for a side stretch. Take a few deep breaths to stretch your left ribs and the side of your body. Walk your hands back to center, then to the left and breathe into the right side of your ribcage.

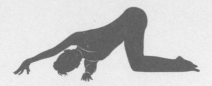

▶ Come up onto all fours, placing your hands slightly wider than shoulder distance apart with your knees under your hips. Do 5 to 10 rounds of **Cat/Cow Pose** (see page 16). Move with the pose by shifting your hips side to side and continuing the spinal curve through your torso.

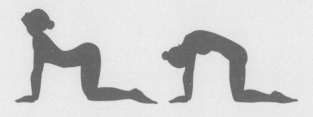

▶ Curl your toes underneath you and press up and back into **Downward-Facing Dog** (see page 20). Press into your hands as you bend your knees and stretch the tops of your thighs up and back. Take 5 deep breaths, and exhale through your mouth to release any tension in your throat and jaw.

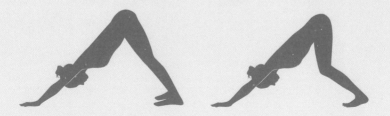

▶ Walk your feet up to your hands, straighten your knees, and allow your upper body to release over your legs into **Forward Fold** (see page 25).

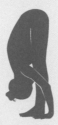

▶ After 3 breaths, bring your hands to your hips, lift your shoulders, and rise up into **Mountain Pose** (see page 34).

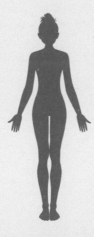

▶ Begin **Sun Salutation A** (see page 45). Stand in **Mountain Pose** with your feet hip distance apart and parallel. As you inhale, reach your arms up to the sky into **Upward Salute** (see page 49). As you exhale, **Forward Fold** and bring your fingers to the earth. As you inhale, bring your fingertips to your shins and move into **Halfway Lift** (see page 29).

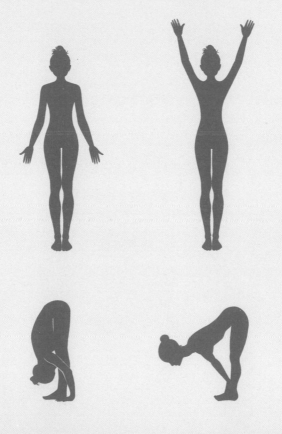

▶ As you exhale, place your palms to the earth shoulder distance apart and step back into **Plank Pose** (see page 36). As you continue to exhale, slowly lower halfway or fully down to the earth into **Four-Limbed Staff Pose** (see page 26). As you inhale, reach your chest forward and up into **Cobra Pose** (see page 18) or **Upward-Facing Dog** (see page 50).

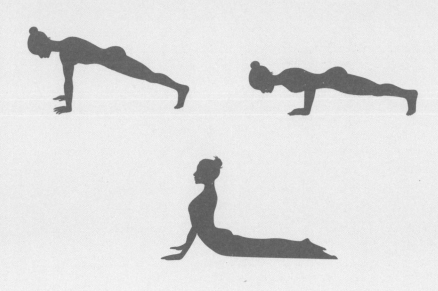

▶ As you exhale, engage your core and reach your hips up and back to come into **Downward-Facing Dog** (see page 20). Take 5 deep breaths. After 5 exhales, step or walk your feet to the front of your mat. Inhale, bring your fingertips to your shins, and lift halfway up into a mini backbend. Exhale into a **Forward Fold** with your fingertips on the earth. Inhale, press through your feet, and reach your arms up into the sky for **Upward Salute**. Exhale and bring your hands to your sides to come back into **Mountain Pose**. Repeat 3 to 5 times. Arrive back in **Mountain Pose** and bring your hands to your heart. Close your eyes and set an intention for your day.

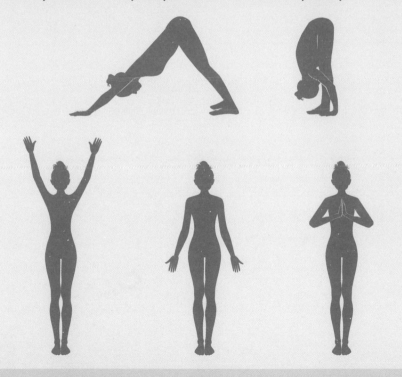

Strong Start

▶ Beginning on all fours, place your forearms on the floor under your elbows, interlace your fingers, and step one foot back at a time to come into **Forearm Plank** (see page 25). Stay for 15 breaths. Lower your knees, place your hands slightly wider than shoulder distance apart, and lift your hips up and back into **Downward-Facing Dog** (see page 20). Stay for 5 breaths.

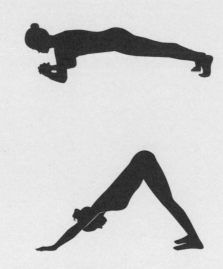

▶ Walk your hands to your feet, then rise up to stand in **Mountain Pose** (see page 34). Begin **Sun Salutation A** (see page 45). As you inhale, reach your arms up to the sky into **Upward Salute** (see page 49). As you exhale, **Forward Fold** (see page 25) and bring your fingers to the earth. As you inhale, bring your fingertips to your shins, and move into **Halfway Lift** (see page 29).

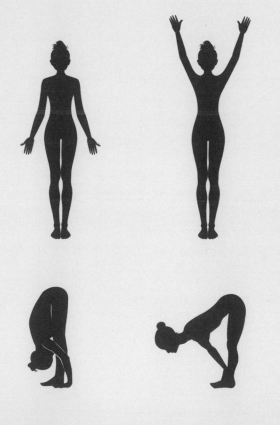

▶ As you exhale, place your palms to the earth shoulder distance apart and step back into **Plank Pose** (see page 36). As you continue to exhale, slowly lower halfway or fully down to the earth into **Four-Limbed Staff Pose** (see page 26). As you inhale, reach your chest forward and up into **Cobra Pose** (see page 18) or **Upward-Facing Dog** (see page 50). As you exhale, engage your core and reach your hips up and back to come into **Downward-Facing Dog**. Take 5 deep breaths.

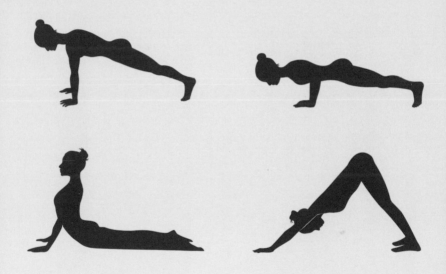

▶ Reach your right leg up and back behind you. As you exhale, draw your right knee to your nose and into **Plank Pose** and pause. Inhale and reach your left leg back up into **Three-Legged Downward-Facing Dog** (see page 48), then draw your knee to your nose and stretch forward into **Plank Pose**. Reach your leg up and back into **Three-Legged Downward-Facing Dog**, then draw your knee to your nose and step your foot between your hands. Turn your back heel on its side and line up your front heel to your back arch.

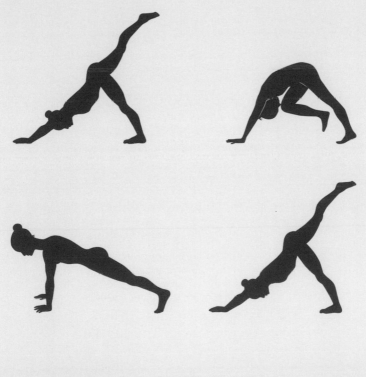

▶ Windmill your arms up to **Warrior 2** (see page 51). Bend your right knee so that it is directly above your ankle and your front thigh is parallel to the floor. Press your left knee wide toward the right side of your mat so that you stretch your outer glute. Press into your back heel and straighten your left leg. Take 8 slow, deep breaths. Bring your hands to the floor and either step back into **Downward-Facing Dog** or take a vinyasa. Repeat this series, beginning with **Plank Pose**, on your left side.

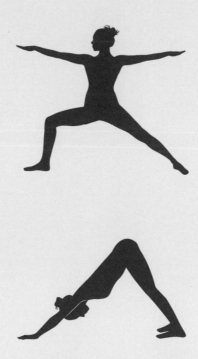

▶ Inhale and reach your right leg up and back into **Three-Legged Downward-Facing Dog**. As you exhale, draw your right knee across your body to your left elbow. Repeat twice. On the third exhale, step your right foot to your right thumb. With your feet hip distance apart and parallel, inhale and reach your arms up to the sky for a **High-Crescent Lunge** (see page 30). Deeply bend your back knee and hover it off the floor as you stretch your arms up. Hold this pose for 10 breaths.

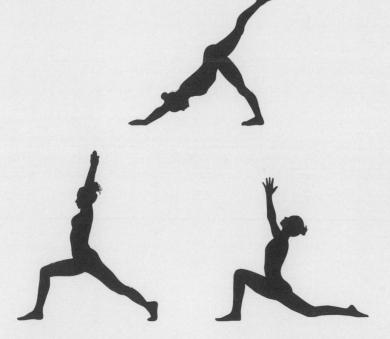

▶ As you exhale, take your hands to the floor, place your left hand under your left shoulder, and reach your right arm up to the sky to come into **Revolved Side Angle Pose** (see page 41). Stay for 5 breaths, lengthening on the inhale and twisting to your right as you exhale. Lower your hand and either step into **Downward-Facing Dog** or take a vinyasa. Repeat the lunge and twist on your other side. From **Downward-Facing Dog**, walk, step or jump your feet up to your hands. Inhale into **Halfway Lift**, and exhale into **Forward Fold**. Inhale and rise all the way up to stand, reaching your arms to the sky. Exhale and bring your hands to your heart for **Mountain Pose**. Close your eyes and take 5 slow, deep breaths, setting your intention for the day.

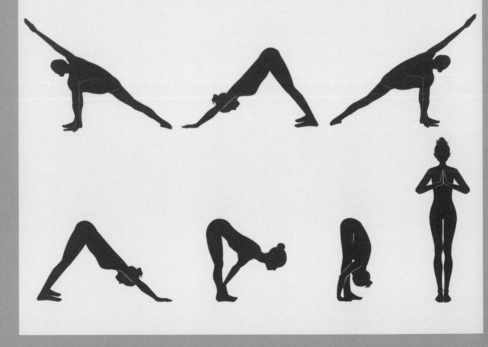

Satisfying Start

▶ Start on your back in **Reclined Mountain Pose** (see page 39) with your knees bent and your feet as wide as your mat. Drop your knees in toward each other and completely relax your hips. Take 10 deep breaths, feeling your body relax into the floor.

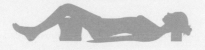

▶ Begin to move your knees from side to side slowly for a variation of an **Abdominal Twist** (see page 14) for about 5 rounds, relaxing your spine as you move.

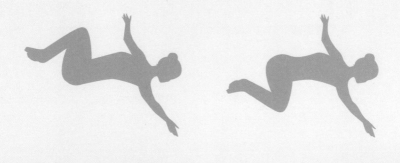

▶ Begin **Pelvic Clock** (see page 35) by bringing your knees completely to one side. Roll over onto that side and come onto all fours with your knees under your hips. Place your elbows under your shoulders, interlace your hands, and take your hips in a big, lazy circle to open your lower back and your shoulders. Move in one direction for about 5 rounds, then change directions.

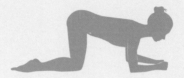

▶ Come onto your hands and begin **Cat/Cow Pose** (see page 16), arching and rounding your spine, for about 10 breaths.

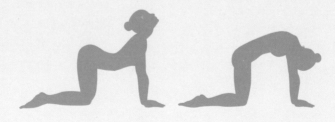

▶ Curl your toes underneath yourself and press up and back into **Downward-Facing Dog** (see page 20). Inhale and come forward into **Plank Pose** (see page 36), then exhale back to **Downward-Facing Dog**. Repeat 5 times.

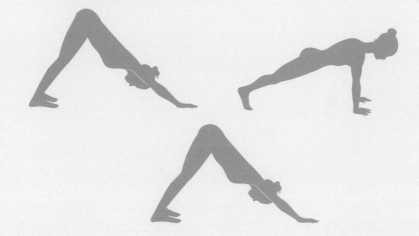

▶ Exhale and lower all the way to the floor. Place your fingers wider than your mat. Perch on your fingertips with your elbows straight above your wrists. As you inhale, draw your head forward and up for **Finger Stand Cobra** (see page 24). As your breathe, move freely, allowing one shoulder to drop forward and then the other, rolling your head and neck to help you fully relax your shoulder muscles. Stay for 5 breaths.

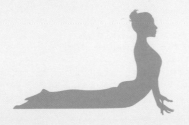

▶ Press up and back into **Downward-Facing Dog**. Walk your hands back to your feet, bend your knees, and bring your hands to your hips. Inhale and slowly lift up into **Mountain Pose** (see page 34). Bring your hands together in front of your heart and take 5 deep breaths to center yourself for the day.

Quick Start

▶ Bring your feet hip distance apart and parallel, bend your knees, and sit back into **Chair Pose** (see page 17). Bring your arms up at an angle, similar to a cactus. Tip your elbows forward slightly and your hands back. Then, claw the air with your fingers and pull down to feel your shoulder blades pull back and your chest lift forward and up. Take 10 breaths, widening your chest and pressing into your heels.

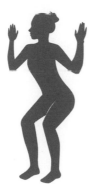
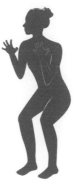

▶ Exhale and **Forward Fold** (see page 25), inhale into **Halfway Lift** (see page 29), then exhale and step back into **Plank Pose** (see page 36). Interlace your hands behind your back, then lift your chest forward and up for **Locust Pose** (see page 32). Tense your core to stabilize your lower back, then lift your legs if you are able. Stay for 5 breaths.

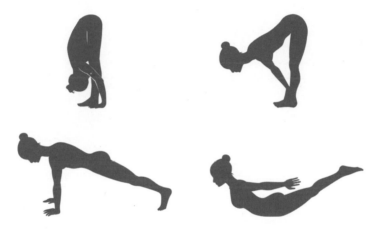

▶ Exhale and press up and back into **Downward-Facing Dog** (see page 20) for 5 breaths. Enhance your stretch by bending one knee and pressing into the opposite heel one side at a time.

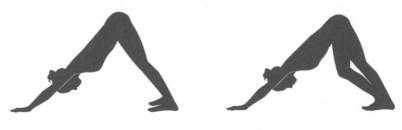

▶ At the end of your exhale, walk, step, or jump your feet to your hands. Inhale into **Halfway Lift**. Exhale and **Forward Fold**, then inhale back to **Chair Pose** (see page 17).

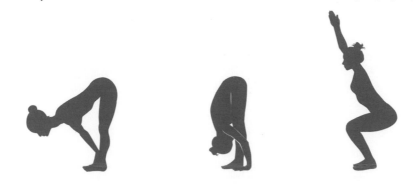

▶ The next two steps are linked together for one side of the body. Sitting low, cross your left thigh over your right, squeezing your legs together for **Eagle Pose** (see page 20). Swing your left arm under your right and either hold onto opposite shoulders or twine your forearms and press your palms together. Take 2 deep breaths, then hinge from your hips to come forward into **Nesting Eagle Pose** (see page 34) with your elbows in front of your knees. Keeping your arms as they are, unwind your legs slowly and extend your left leg toward the back of your mat.

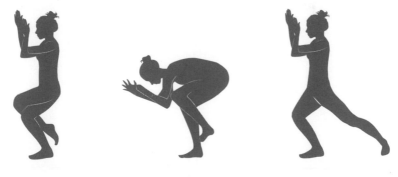

▶ Step into **High-Crescent Lunge** (see page 30). Ensure your feet are hip distance apart and parallel, then release your arms and stretch them upward. Lower into your legs, bring your front thigh to a 90° angle, then press up through the ball of your back foot. Press through your feet as your reach up through your arms for 5 breaths.

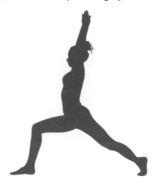

▶ As you exhale, bring your left hand to the floor under your left shoulder and reach your right arm up to the sky for **Revolved Side Angle Pose** (see page 41). Sweep your arm back by your hip and rotate your arm and shoulder in wide circles for 5 rounds. Place your hands on blocks directly under your shoulders. As you inhale, drop your hips forward for a lunge, then exhale and pull your hips back and bend your torso over your front leg. Move forward and back to stretch your hamstrings. Hold this pose for 5 rounds, gently moving your hips back and forth.

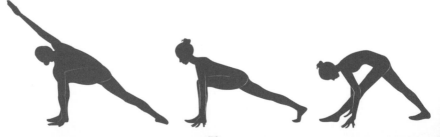

▶ Step forward to the front of your mat and inhale into **Halfway Lift**. Exhale and **Forward Fold**. Inhale to **Chair Pose**, and repeat this flow on the opposite side. Step forward to the front of your mat, bend your knees, and release the weight of your upper body down to the floor for **Forward Fold**. You can let your body sway or hold onto opposite elbows.

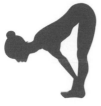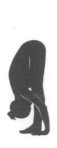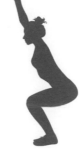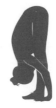

▶ Bring your hands to your hips, bend your knees, and slowly rise up into **Mountain Pose** (see page 34). Bring your hands together in front of your heart and set an intention for your day.

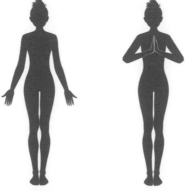

Breath-Infused Start

▶ Start in **Mountain Pose** (see page 34) with your feet hip distance apart and parallel. Bring your left hand over your heart and your right hand over your left and feel your heartbeat. Take 5 deep breaths into your chest. Lower your hands to your side and press down through your feet. As you inhale, reach your arms wide and up, press your palms together, and look up at your fingers. As you exhale, slowly drag your pressed palms down through the center of your body. At about your navel, interlace your hands and press your palms toward the floor. Follow your hands with your gaze. Repeat 5 to 10 times.

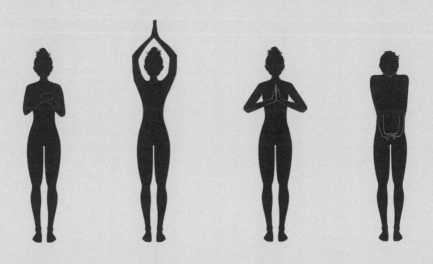

▶ Begin **Half Sun Salutation** (see page 28) by inhaling and reaching your arms up to the sky for **Upward Salute** (see page 49). Exhale and bend your knees slightly into **Forward Fold** (see page 25). Inhale into **Halfway Lift** (see page 29). Exhale back into **Forward Fold**. Inhale, rise up, and reach your arms up into **Upward Salute**. Exhale and bring your hands to your sides. Repeat 4 times, focusing on the connection of your movement with your breath.

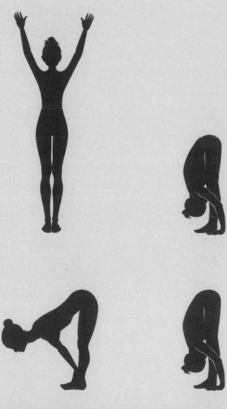

▶ To begin **Sun Salutation B** (see page 46) with a high lunge, bend your knees, then inhale and reach your arms up to the sky for **Chair Pose** (see page 17). Exhale into **Forward Fold**. On the inhale, come into **Halfway Lift**.

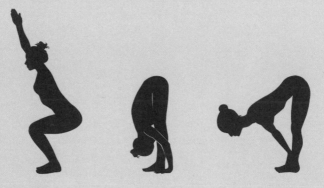

▶ Exhale, step back into **Plank Pose** (see page 36) and lower down into **Four-Limbed Staff Pose** (see page 26). Inhale into a backbend, then exhale to **Downward-Facing Dog** (see page 20).

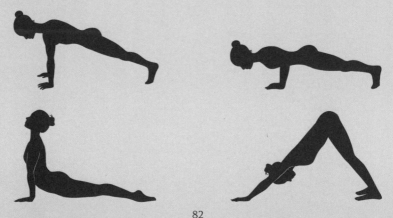

▶ Step your right foot to your right thumb, lower your back knee, if you desire, and reach your arms up into **High-Crescent Lunge** (see page 30). As you exhale, lower your hands to the earth and step back into a vinyasa or into **Downward-Facing Dog** for 5 deep breaths. Step your left foot to your left thumb and inhale to rise up into **High-Crescent Lunge** on the other side, and repeat the sequence.

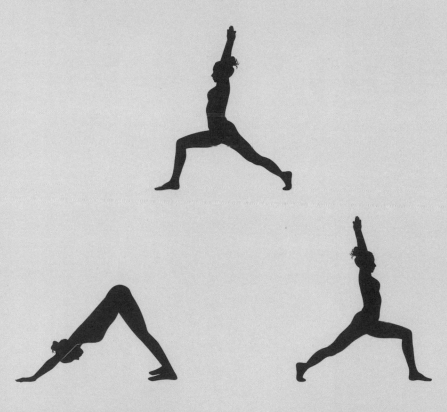

▶ At the end of your last exhale in **Downward-Facing Dog**, walk, step, or jump your feet forward. Inhale into **Halfway Lift**, then exhale into **Forward Fold**. Inhale and bend your knees into **Chair Pose**. Exhale into **Mountain Pose**. Repeat the sequence, including the side switch, two more times, focusing on linking your breathing with your movement.

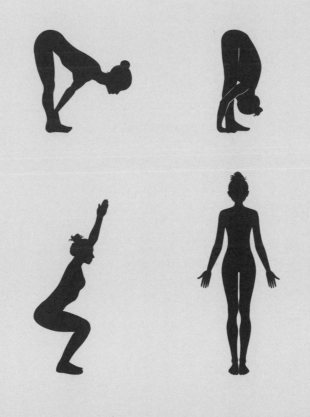

▶ Stand in **Mountain Pose** with your left hand on your heart and right hand over your left, feeling your heartbeat and your breathing. Take 3 deep breaths to set your intention for the day.

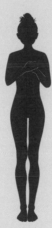

Midday Pick-Me-Ups

WARRIOR STRONG

▶ Stand in **Mountain Pose** (see page 34) in the middle of your mat, facing the long side. Bring your hands together in front of your heart, closing your eyes to bring your attention inward. Take 5 long, deep breaths. Bend your knees, sit your hips back, reach your arms forward and up, and come into **Chair Pose** (see page 17). Press your heels down and bring your inner thighs slightly back and down. Then, angle your tailbone down slightly to lift through your lower belly. As you send your hips back, stretch the sides of your waist. Then, stretch all the way through your fingertips. Stay for 10 breaths.

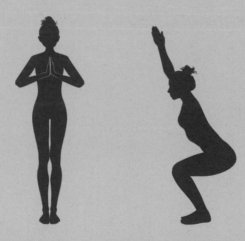

▶ Open your eyes and step your feet out wide. Rotate your right thigh, shin, and foot so that they they face the short side of your mat. Turn your back toes in slightly, then bend your right knee and move down into **Warrior 2** (see page 51). Lift your arms to shoulder height and stretch through your arms. Sit down onto your right thigh until it is parallel to the floor. Wrap your right glute underneath you as you bring your left thigh straight and press through your back heel. Stay here for 10 long, slow breaths, allowing the slow, strong burn of this pose to build your energy. Repeat on the other side.

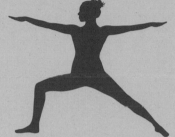

▶ Turn both feet toward the long end of your mat and bring your hands onto your hips. Inhale to lift your chest, and as you exhale, hinge over your pelvis into **Wide Legged Forward Fold** (see page 52). You can either bring your hands to the floor (or blocks) for support, or interlace your hands behind your back and lift your arms to the sky to add a shoulder opening. Press into your feet as you work to straighten your legs and release your upper body. Stay for 5 breaths. Bring your hands to your hips, soften your knees, and inhale to rise up.

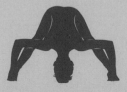

▶ Turn your right thigh and foot toward the short end of your mat again, and bring your left toes slightly in. Bend your right knee square (as in **Warrior 2**), then hinge from your pelvis to send your tailbone toward your back heel and bring your right forearm onto your right thigh for **Side Angle Pose** (see page 41). Keep your knee directly over the center of your foot by tensing your right glute, then, turn your pelvis and chest to the left and reach your left arm up to the sky. You can also keep your right elbow on your knee, bring your elbow to the inside of your knee, or hover your elbow above your thigh. Stay for 10 breaths. Repeat on your left side.

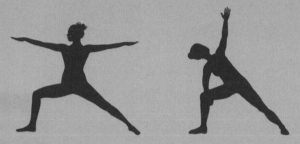

▶ Return to **Mountain Pose**, feeling the strength of your legs and your connection to the earth. Take 3 deep breaths to anchor yourself.

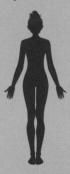

Quick and Breezy Flow

▶ Begin in **Mountain Pose** (see page 34). Bring your hands to your heart and take 3 deep, clearing breaths. Begin **Half Sun Salutation** (see page 28) by inhaling. Reach your arms up to the sky for **Upward Salute** (see page 49). Exhale into **Forward Fold** (see page 25). Inhale into **Halfway Lift** (see page 29). Exhale back into **Forward Fold**. Inhale, rise up, and reach your arms up for **Upward Salute**. Exhale and bring your hands back down to your sides. Repeat 4 more times.

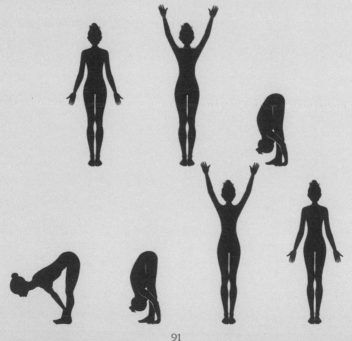

▶ Move into **Sun Salutation A** (see page 45) with a flowing lunge and half split by inhaling and reaching your arms up to the sky. Exhale into a **Forward Fold**. Inhale and raise into **Halfway Lift**. Exhale and step your left foot back behind you and lower your back knee down. Keeping your hands on the floor (or on blocks) by your front foot, inhale and drop your hips forward. Lift your chest forward, exhale, and slide your hips back into a **Forward Fold** over your front thigh. Move between these two movements on your inhale, and exhale at least 5 times, enjoying the fluidity through your shoulders, spine, and hips.

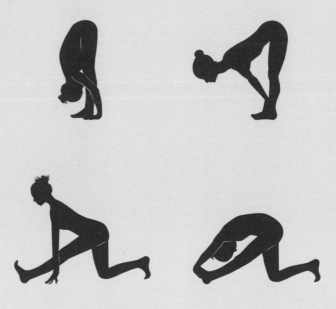

▶ After 5 to 7 rounds, step back to the front of your mat, step your right foot back, and repeat through your opposite side. Exhale and step back into **Downward-Facing Dog** (see page 20).

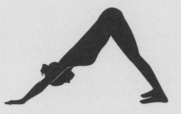

▶ From **Downward-Facing Dog**, stretch your right leg back and up into **Three-Legged Downward-Facing Dog** (see page 48). Open your hips, bend your left knee, then draw your right knee into your belly and make five giant circles with your right knee to take your hip through its full range of motion.

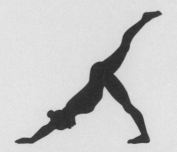

▶ Stretch your right leg straight back and inhale. As you exhale, draw your knee into your nose and shift forward into **Plank Pose** (see page 36). Inhale and stretch your leg back into **Three-Legged Downward-Facing Dog**, then exhale and draw your knee to your nose. Inhale and stretch your leg back, exhale and draw your knee to your nose, and then place your right foot between your hands.

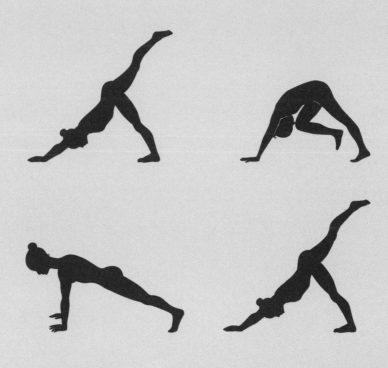

▶ Turn your back heel down parallel to the edge of your mat and rise up into **Warrior 2** (see page 51). Keeping your front knee over your front heel, inhale and reach your right arm up to side stretch into **Exalted Warrior Pose** (see page 22). As you exhale, shift your hips back, bring your right forearm onto your thigh, and sweep your top arm over your ear for **Side Angle Pose** (see page 42). Alternate between these two shapes for 5 to 7 rounds. On your final exhale, take your hands all the way to the floor, step back into **Downward-Facing Dog**, and repeat on your left side.

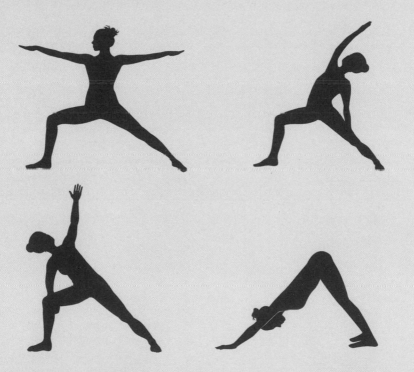

▶ Take your hands all the way to the floor. Inhale to step forward to the front of your mat and come into a **Halfway Lift**. Exhale into **Forward Fold**. Inhale to rise all the way up and stand with your arms overhead for **Upward Salute**, then exhale and bring your hands to your heart into **Mountain Pose**. Close your eyes and take 5 slow, deep breaths.

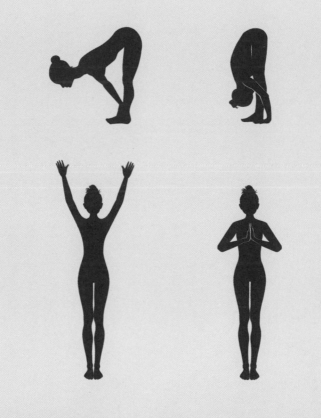

QUICK CORE CONNECTION

▶ Begin by lying on your back in **Reclined Mountain Pose** (see page 39) with your knees bent and your feet hip distance apart. Take a few deep breaths to clear your mind.

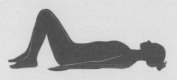

▶ Draw your knees into your chest for **Knees-to-Chest Pose** (see page 31) and slide your hands behind your head. Relax your shoulders, point your elbows up to the sky, and relax your head into your hands. Keeping your lower back pressed to your mat, bring your legs into **Tabletop Pose** (see page 47) with your knees above your pelvis and inhale. As you exhale, draw your left elbow toward your outer right knee. Inhale and come back to center with your head off the floor. As you exhale, twist your right elbow to your outer left knee. Repeat 10 times each side. Then, draw your knees into your chest and take a few deep belly breaths.

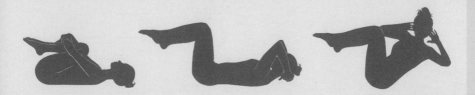

▶ Roll over onto one side and come onto your forearms and your knees to prepare for **Forearm Plank** (see page 25). Place your elbows under your knees with your hands interlaced, then step one foot back at a time to straighten your legs. Bring your lower ribs up into your body and press your shoulders away from your ears. Stay for 15 breaths.

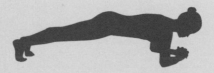

▶ Come down onto your knees, place your hands under your shoulders, and press up and back into **Downward-Facing Dog** (see page 20) for 5 breaths.

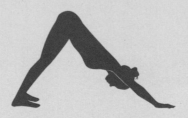

▶ Inhale and lift your left leg high. As you exhale, draw your knee to your nose, shift forward, and round your spine. Inhale and stretch your leg back into **Three-Legged Downward-Facing Dog** (see page 48); as you exhale, shift forward and round your body. Repeat twice more, then step your right foot up to your right thumb and lower your back knee down.

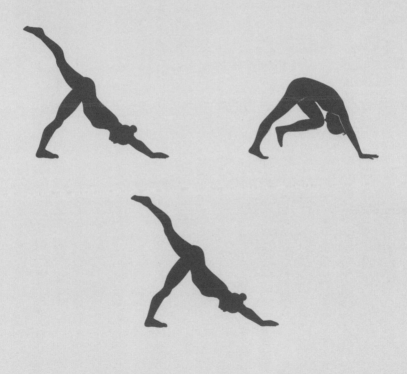

▶ Bring your hands together at the center of your chest, inhale, then exhale and bring your left elbow to your outer right knee for **Revolved Side Angle Pose** (see page 41). If you want, you can lift your back knee up to deepen the pose. Inhale and lengthen, then exhale and twist for 5 rounds of breathing. As you inhale, untwist and bring your hands to the floor, then step back into **Downward-Facing Dog**. Repeat on your opposite side.

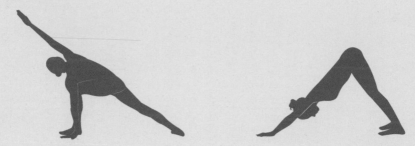

▶ Walk your feet to your hands. With your feet hip distance apart, hold your opposite elbows and **Forward Fold** (see page 25). Hold for 10 breaths. Then, release your arms and slowly roll up through your spine. Stand in **Mountain Pose** (see page 34) for 5 slow breaths.

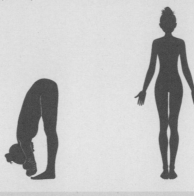

WONDER WALL

For this practice, you will need a clear space at a wall. If you are using a mat, place the short end of your mat at the wall.

▶ Place your hands at hip height on the wall, and step back into an L-shaped variation of **Warrior 3** (see page 51). Ensure your hands are shoulder distance apart. Press into your hands, bend your knees slightly, and push your hips back into the center of the room to lengthen your spine. Keeping your spine straight, begin to straighten your legs and hold for 10 breaths. Then, walk your feet back toward the wall and stand up.

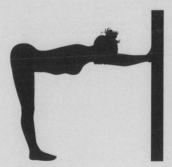

▶ Turn around with your back to the wall and place your feet about shin distance from the wall. Lean your hips back into the wall. Bend your knees and sit down into **Chair Pose** (see page 17). Press your heels straight down into your mat, being careful not to slide them forward. Reach your arms forward at shoulder height. Keeping your low ribs pressed back into the wall, press your shoulders back and reach your arms straight upward. Hold for 10 breaths, then lean forward to stand up.

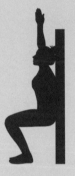

▶ Turn to face the long side of your mat with your left foot at the wall. Place your feet wide apart for **Warrior 2** (see page 51). Turn your left toes forward slightly. From the top of your right thigh, rotate your front leg until your toes point toward the short end of your mat and your ankle, shin, and thigh are aligned. Keeping your back heel pressed against the wall, bend your right knee into a right angle. Press your feet apart as you reach your arms wide. Take 10 breaths, then switch sides.

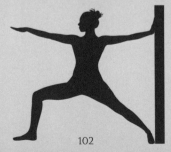

▶ Place your hands at hip height at the wall again and return to the L-shaped pose variation of **Warrior 3**. Press your hands into the wall and keep your spine straight. Bring your legs together and reach your right foot back toward the center of the room. Keep your arms straight and your hips squared. Stay for 10 slow breaths on each side.

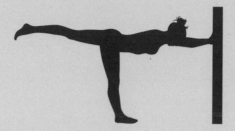

▶ Walk your feet slowly forward and rise up into **Mountain Pose** (see page 34). Take 5 breaths and feel how refreshed your hips and shoulders are.

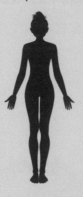

Revitalize Your Feet

▶ Begin on all fours. Tuck your toes underneath you, then sit back on your heels for a toe stretch in **Hero's Pose** (see page 30). To decrease the intensity of the stretch, you can sit on a block or lift your pelvis up slightly. If possible, allow your body weight to sink down onto your heels, relaxing your front ribs in and your shoulders down. Bring your hands together in front of your heart and take 5 to 10 deep breaths.

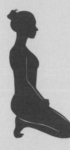

▶ Exhale, come onto all fours, point your toes, and tap the tops of your feet to your mat. Begin 5 to 10 rounds of **Cat/Cow Pose** (see page 16) to open your shoulders and hips.

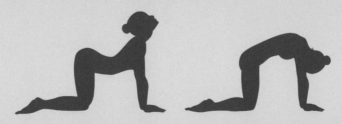

▶ Press up and back into **Downward-Facing Dog** (see page 20) for 5 to 10 breaths.

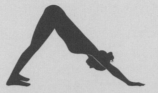

▶ Walk your feet to your hands and **Forward Fold** (see page 25). Hold for 5 breaths.

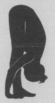

▶ Roll up into **Mountain Pose** (see page 34). Shift your weight side to side, then forward and backward to feel connected to the earth.

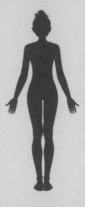

▶ Bring your feet together. Sit down deeply into **Chair Pose** (see page 17) with your weight in your heels, and bring your hands together in front of your heart. Squeeze your legs together. Keeping your knees and thighs pressed in, lift your left foot off the floor and balance on your right foot for 5 slow breaths. Repeat on the opposite side.

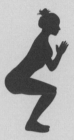

▶ Stand in **Mountain Pose** with your feet together and your hands on your hips. Use your hands to keep your pelvis squared forward, then turn your right thigh out and bring your foot to your shin or upper inner thigh for **Tree Pose** (see page 49). If you feel stable, reach your arms up overhead. Press down into your standing foot as you stretch up through the sides of your body. Take 5 breaths, then repeat on the opposite side.

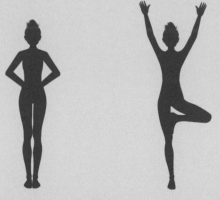

▶ The next four poses are linked together in a flow. Bend you knees and sit back into a deep **Chair Pose**. Inhale to lengthen your spine. As you exhale, bring your left elbow to the outside of your right knee for **Revolved Chair Pose** (see page 40). Inhale to lengthen, exhale to twist. Maintaining your twist, keep your knees aligned. With your knees pressed together, lift your left foot off the floor. Press your chest forward as you slowly stretch your left leg back toward the back of your mat. Keep your upper body low.

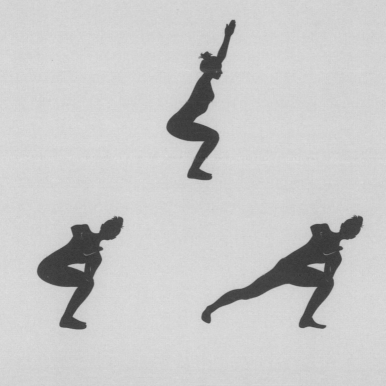

▶ Step back into **Revolved Side Angle Pose** (see page 41). Pressing strongly into your feet, squeeze your legs together. Inhale and rise up into **High-Crescent Lunge** (see page 30). Hold for 5 breaths.

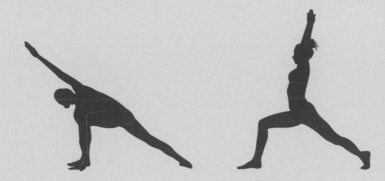

▶ Bring your hands to the floor, bend your front knee, and step forward into **Standing Split** (see page 44). Press into your right heel and begin to stretch your right leg straight. Stretch your left leg up and into the air, rolling your outer left hip down to keep your hips square. For an extra balance challenge, lift one or both hands off the floor and bring them to your right calf. Take 5 breaths.

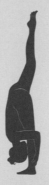

▶ Press into your right foot, bend your right knee, and draw your left knee into your chest. Bring your hands together in front of your heart and begin to stand up. Cross your left ankle over your right knee and sit your hips back for **One-Legged Chair Pose** (see page 35). Press your hips back and your chest forward for 5 breaths. Stand up, release your foot to the floor, and come into **Mountain Pose**. Shake out your legs as needed. Then, repeat the series on your opposite side.

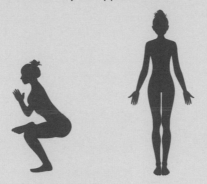

▶ Once finished, stand in **Mountain Pose** with your hands at your heart, feeling the connection of your feet into the floor. Take 5 deep breaths.

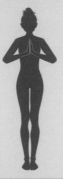

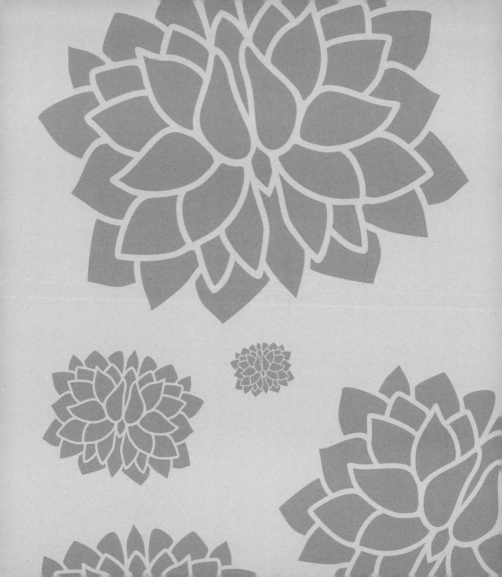

Evening Unwinds

For an Active Mind

▶ Face the front of your mat and stand in **Mountain Pose** (see page 34). Bring your hands together in front of your heart and focus inward. Take 3 long breaths, focusing on the exhale. Open your eyes and reach your arms to the sky to begin 3 rounds of **Sun Salutation A** (see page 45). Focus on breathing fully and staying present through each transition. As you inhale, reach your arms up to the sky into **Upward Salute** (see page 49). As you exhale, **Forward Fold** (see page 25) and bring your fingers to the earth. As you inhale, bring your fingertips to your shins, and move into **Halfway Lift** (see page 29).

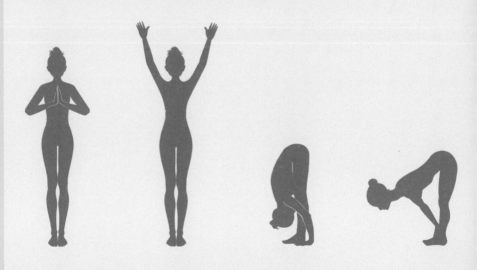

▶ As you exhale, place your palms to the earth shoulder distance apart and step back into **Plank Pose** (see page 36). As you continue to exhale, slowly lower halfway or fully down to the earth into **Four-Limbed Staff Pose** (see page 26). As you inhale, reach your chest forward and up into **Cobra Pose** (see page 18) or **Upward-Facing Dog** (see page 50). As you exhale, engage your core and reach your hips up and back to come into **Downward-Facing Dog** (see page 20). Take 5 deep breaths.

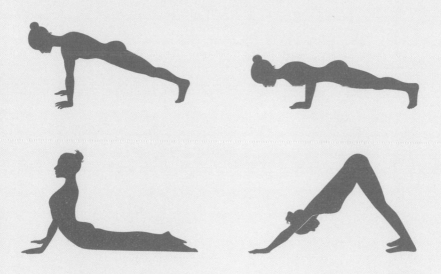

▶ From your final **Downward-Facing Dog**, step your right foot up to your right thumb. Bring your hands to your front thigh and rise up to **High-Crescent Lunge** (see page 30). Reach your arms up into a large V. Sit down deeply onto your front leg, pressing into your back toes to straighten your back leg. As you press down into your feet, reach up through your arms to stretch your whole body. Stay for 5 slow breaths, then press your hands to the floor and either take a vinyasa or move straight to **Downward-Facing Dog**. Repeat on your left side.

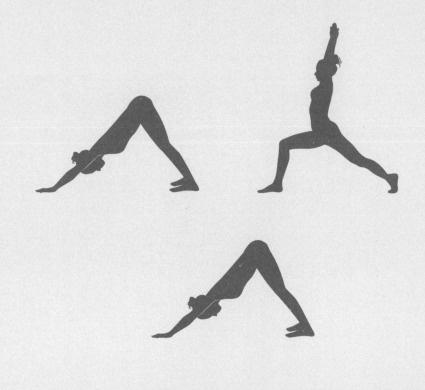

▶ From **Downward-Facing Dog**, inhale forward into **Plank Pose** (see page 36) and lower all the way down onto your belly. Keeping your lower ribs on your mat, stretch each leg back and press the tops of your feet down. Place your hands wider than your mat and position your elbows above your wrists. Inhale, bringing your chest forward and up into **Finger Stand Cobra Pose** (see page 24). Move freely in this pose, rolling your shoulders, head, and neck to relax your upper body. Hold for 5 breaths.

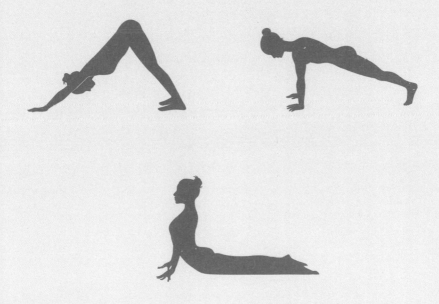

▶ Exhale, lower down, and flip onto your back. Cross your right ankle over your left knee and draw your left knee into your chest to come into **Eye of the Needle Pose** (see page 24). Staying conscious of your breathing, allow your right hip to settle toward your body. Close your eyes and rest your head on the floor. Take 10 deep breaths, then slowly change sides.

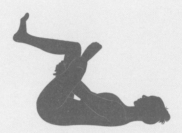

▶ Staying on your back, draw your knees into your chest and bring your shins perpendicular to the floor. Hold on to your shins or outer feet and gently draw your knees out to the side for **Happy Baby** (see page 29). Stay for 10 breaths. Feel free to roll gently side to side.

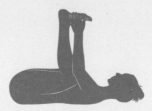

▶ Stretch your legs out straight and bring one hand to your belly and the other hand to your heart for **Corpse Pose** (see page 18). If your mind is still active, then use the connection of your hands to your body to focus your attention to the easy rise and fall of your chest. Allow your body to completely relax into the floor. Stay as long as you wish.

Satisfying Hip Opening

▶ Begin in **Child's Pose** (see page 17) with your knees out wide and take 10 deep breaths. Allow your pelvis to get heavier against your heels and deliberately release your body weight downward. Relax your shoulders, arms, and torso.

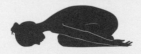

▶ Come onto all fours and take 5 to 10 rounds of **Cat/Cow Pose** (see page 16) to release any tension through your spine. Feel free to roll your shoulders and shift your hips from side to side. Step your right foot forward into **Low Lunge** (see page 33). If you are able, you can allow your knee to move in front of your ankle to stretch through your calf. Be careful of overextending your knee. Keep your hands on your front thigh, or reach your arms up to the sky to stretch the side of your waist. Squeeze your right glute to stretch the front of your hip. Take 5 deep breaths, then change sides.

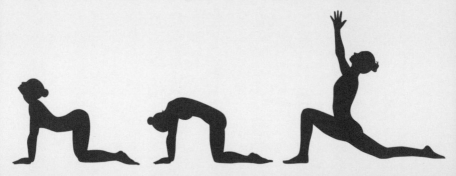

▶ Sit on your right hip and bring your right shin parallel with the short end of your mat. Place your left shin parallel to the long edge of your mat similar to the **90/90 Pose** (see page 14) and inhale. As you exhale, hinge over your front thigh to stretch your outer hip. For this variation on **Pigeon Pose** (see page 36), keep your right hip anchored to the earth and slide your left leg back behind you until you feel a deep stretch through your outer right hip. Stay for 10 to 15 breaths. You can switch out **Pigeon Pose** with **Eye of the Needle Pose** (see page 24), depending on your comfort level.

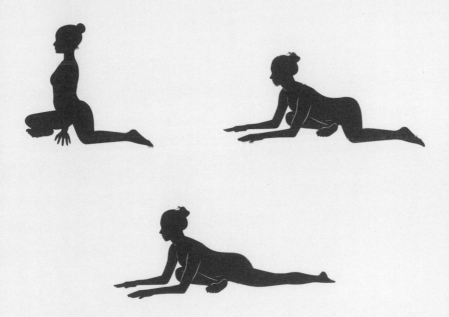

▶ Before going to the other side, walk your hands back up so you are sitting, then swing your left leg up and over your right to stack your knees for **Cow Face Pose** (see page 19). Press through your tailbone, place your heels equidistant from the sides of your pelvis, and fold forward over your legs until you feel a stretch through your outer hip. If desired, you can move into **Reclined Cow Face Pose** (see page 38) instead. Take 10 to 15 breaths, then repeat on the opposite side.

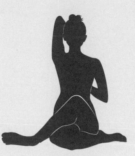

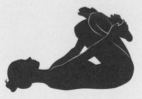

▶ Turn toward the long end of your mat and bring your knees wide apart for **Frog Pose** (see page 26). Rest onto your forearms. Align your ankles with your knees, keeping your pelvis over your knees. Then, shift your hips back slightly to stretch your inner thighs. Depending on your body, you may bring your heels slightly closer together, or support your pelvis and stomach with a bolster or pillow. Stay for 15 breaths, allowing gravity to gently open your inner legs. You can switch out **Frog Pose** with **Happy Baby** (see page 29), depending on your comfort level.

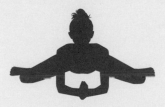

▶ Come to lay on your back for **Corpse Pose** (see page 18), allowing your body to completely release to the earth.

Shoulder Release

For this practice, it is best to have a strap or a towel on hand, as well as a block or book for support.

▶ Come into **Child's Pose** (see page 17) with your hips on your heels. If your forehead doesn't reach the floor, use a block or a book to support your head and release any tension through your head and neck. Relax your jaw. Take 5 slow, deep breaths, relaxing your back and shoulders as you exhale.

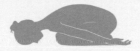

▶ Lift up partway, and thread your right arm underneath your left, coming into **Supported Child's Pose with Twist** (see page 47). You can continue to rest your head on a block or book, if desired, as well as use a block or towel to support your hips. Take 5 breaths, then change sides.

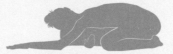

▶ Come onto all fours and take 5 to 10 rounds of **Cat/Cow Pose** (see page 16) to relax your spine.

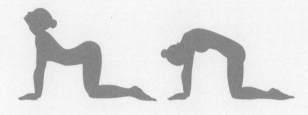

▶ Come back to all fours and press into **Downward-Facing Dog** (see page 20) for a few breaths to stretch the backs of your legs.

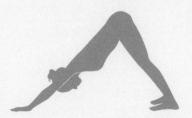

► Step your right foot to your right hand and lower your back knee down for a **Low Lunge** (see page 33). Reach your left arm overhead and use your right hand to turn your outer arm forward. Bend your left elbow and bring your left hand to the middle of your back to add a triceps stretch. Relax your front ribs and bring your hips forward. Take 5 slow breaths, then lower your hands and change sides.

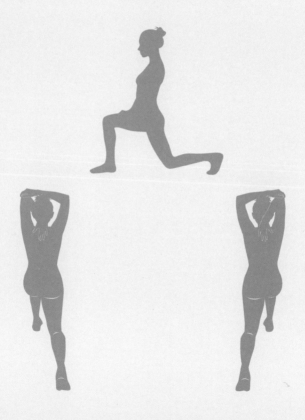

▶ Step your right foot between your hands, turn you back heel down and align your front heel with your back foot's arch. Keep your right knee over your ankle and rise up into **Warrior 2** (see page 51). Interlace your hands behind your back. If this is too tight for your shoulders, then hold a towel with your palms facing forward. Bend your elbows and draw your upper arms back. Keeping your chest wide, stretch your arms straight. Breathe into your upper chest. Take 5 breaths, then release your hands downward and repeat on the opposite side with a different interlock of your fingers.

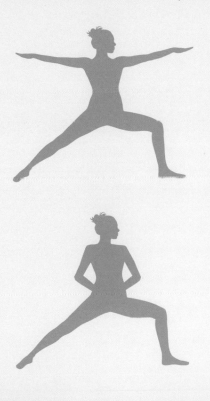

▶ Standing at the front of your mat in **Mountain Pose** (see page 34), hold your strap slightly wider than shoulder distance apart. For this shoulder flossing exercise, keep your arms straight, but feel free to slide your hands as wide as you need along the strap to facilitate movement. As you inhale, lift your arms up and overhead. Continue to pull the strap apart as you reach your arms all the way behind you. Inhale to lift the strap up to sky; exhale as you bring your arms to your sides. Repeat 5 times.

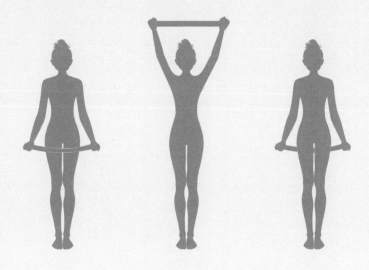

▶ Lay on your stomach and extend your right arm out to the side level with your shoulder. Keep your palm flat. Use your left hand to roll onto your right side into an intense shoulder stretch. For a deeper stretch, you can turn your left knee upward and press your foot down behind your right knee. You can keep your left hand on the floor in front of your chest to support you, or place it behind your back. Stay for 5 breaths, then change sides.

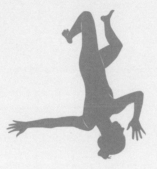

▶ Lay on your back in **Corpse Pose** (see page 18) and allow your body to relax into the floor.

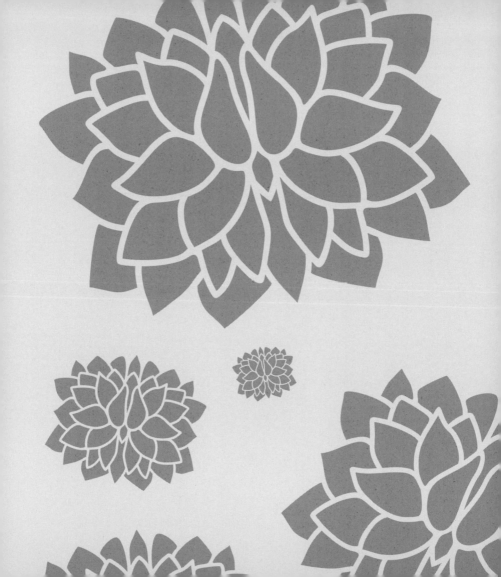

Soulful Self-Care

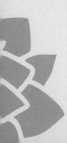

FOR STRENGTH AND RESILIENCE

▶ Come into **Extended Child's Pose** (see page 23) by taking your hips to your heels. Rest your forehead on your hands, a book, a block, or the floor. Relax your face. Exhale, allow your body to relax fully into the floor, releasing the tension in your head and neck. Pressing your left hip back and down, walk your hands to the right side of your mat for **Thread the Needle Pose** (see page 48). Take a few deep breaths to expand your chest and stretch your side. Tilt your chest up or down, depending on which provides the deepest stretch. Repeat on the opposite side.

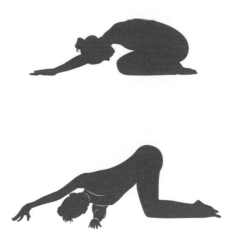

► Keeping your face relaxed, bring yourself onto all fours. Inhale and reach your right leg back and your left arm forward. Then, draw your right knee to your stomach and your left elbow to your knee as you exhale. Begin 5 to 10 rounds of **Extended Cat Pose** (see page 22) on both sides, timing your breathing with your movement as you stretch and retract. It's okay to wobble.

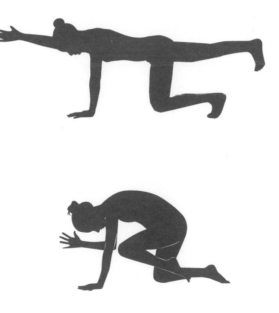

▶ Press your hands down onto your mat, curl your toes underneath yourself, and hover your knees off the floor in a modified **Plank Pose** (see page 36). Focus on working your core as you draw your bottom ribs in and lengthen your tailbone downward. Stay for 10 to 15 breaths to feel the strength of your arms and core. It is alright if this pose leaves you shaking.

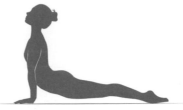

▶ Rest in **Child's Pose** (see page 17) and take 5 deep breaths. Bring your forearms to the floor with your elbows beneath your shoulders and interlace your hands together. Stretch one leg back at a time to come into **Forearm Plank** (see page 25). If desired, you can lower your knees down for additional support. Press into your forearms as you draw your bottom ribs in and widen your shoulders back. Stay for 10 to 20 breaths, focusing on the power behind this pose. Rest in **Child's Pose** (see page 17) and take 10 slow, deep breaths, allowing your body to relax.

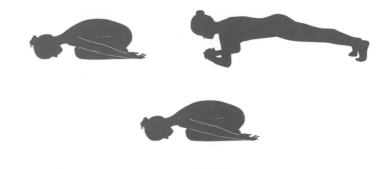

▶ Sit into **Hero's Pose** (see page 30), bring your hands together in front of your heart, and bow your head to your hands, taking a moment to acknowledge your own strength and resilience.

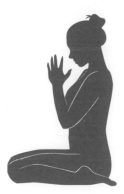

For New Moms

▶ Stand in **Mountain Pose** (see page 34) with your hands at your heart and take 3 deep, clearing breaths, becoming aware of any tension held in your body. Begin **Half Sun Salutation** (see page 28) by inhaling and reaching your arms up and overhead for **Upward Salute** (see page 49). As you exhale, bend your knees and come into **Forward Fold** (see page 25). Inhale to come into **Halfway Lift** (see page 29) and roll your shoulders back and out. As you exhale, move into **Forward Fold** and relax your head and neck. Inhale to rise back up, bringing your arms out wide for **Upward Salute**. As you exhale, bring your hands to your sides. Repeat 3 times, focusing on your breathing to help relax your body.

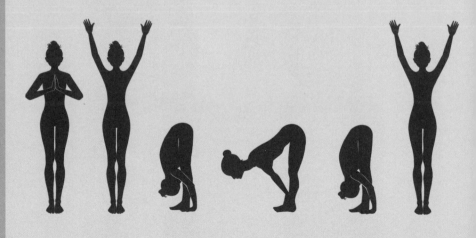

▶ Inhale and bring your arms up. Exhale into **Forward Fold**, come up into **Halfway Lift**, then step your left leg back and lower your back knee down for a **Low Lunge** (see page 33). Place your right hand on your thigh, then stretch your left arm upward. Stretch your side by reaching your left arm over to the right. You can stay in this side stretch, or turn your chest forward and down toward your front thigh to create a deep lower back stretch through the left side of your body. Hold the stretch for 5 to 10 breaths.

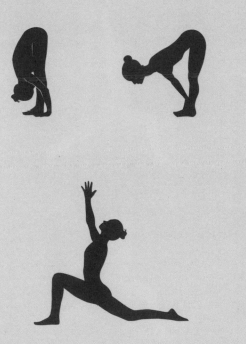

► Place your hands on the floor, lift your back knee, and reach your arms up to come into **High-Crescent Lunge** (see page 30). Interlace your hands behind your back and draw your upper arms backward to bring your chest forward and up. Press your inner legs toward each other and lengthen your tailbone downward to strengthen your pelvic floor. Take 5 deep breaths to open your upper chest and release your shoulders. Bring your hands to the floor and step forward. Then, step your right leg back and repeat this flow on the opposite side.

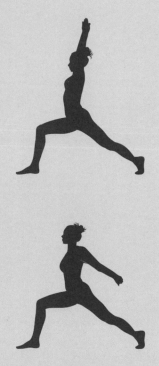

▶ Turn toward the long end of your mat and place your feet wide apart. Turn your right thigh forward and point your toes toward the front of your mat. Tilt your back toes forward slightly. Bend your front knee to a right angle and come into **Warrior 2** (see page 51). Inhale and lift your right arm up to come into **Goddess Pose** (see page 27). Press your weight into your legs, tilt your tailbone downward, and breathe deeply into your core for 5 breaths. Straighten your legs and repeat on the opposite side

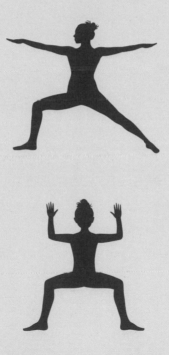

▶ Step to the front of your mat. Inhale and lift your chest. As you exhale, **Forward Fold**. Hold onto your opposite elbows and allow the weight of your upper body to release toward the earth. Shake your head a few times to release your head, neck, and jaw. Allow yourself 3 yawn-like movements to relax your facial muscles. After a few breaths, change the crossing of your arms. Release your arms and slowly roll up to a standing position. Place your hands on your heart in **Mountain Pose** and thank yourself for creating some space and time to nourish your body.

For Anxiety

▶ Begin in **Child's Pose** (see page 17) and take a few deep breaths. If you feel too jittery for child's pose, move straight into **Cat/Cow Pose** (see page 16). Bring your attention to the physical sensations of your body and your breathing.

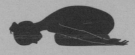

▶ Get onto all fours for **Cat/Cow Pose**. Focus on the connection of your body to the earth. Take 5 to 10 breaths.

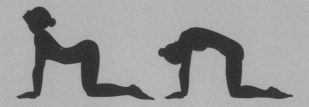

► Step your right foot to your right hand and bring your hands onto your front thigh for **Low Lunge** (see page 33). Press your thighs together. Interlace your hands and press your palms flat. Relax your shoulders and press your palms upward. Take 5 breaths, then lower your hands and repeat on the other side. Bring your hands to the floor, lift your back knee, then turn your back heel parallel to the back of your mat. Align your front heel with your back arch. Keep your right knee over your right ankle.

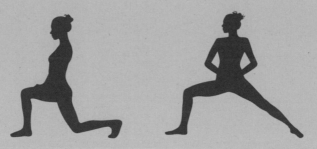

► Place your right forearm on your right thigh and bring your left hand to your left hip for **Side Angle Pose** (see page 42). Pull your outer right hip back towards your back foot and turn your chest to the side of your mat. Reach upward with your left arm. Take 10 breaths, then bring your hands to the floor and change sides.

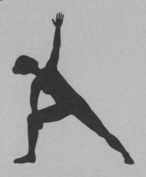

▶ Stand at the front of your mat with your feet and legs together. Bend your knees and sit your hips back into **Chair Pose** (see page 17). Anchor into your heels and lean back. Reach your arms forward and relax your shoulders outward. Stay for 10 slow breaths. To move into **Forward Fold** (see page 25), release your upper body forward over your legs. Bring your feet hip distance apart and take 5 deep breaths to let go of any tension and stress in your body.

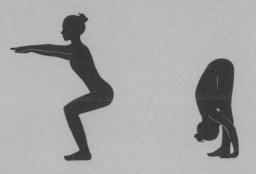

▶ Step back into **Plank Pose** (see page 36), then lower down to your belly. Place your pelvis and legs onto the floor, then interlace your hands behind your back.

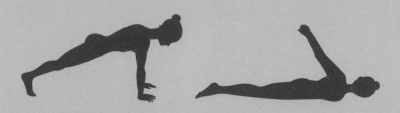

▶ Roll your shoulders, then lift your chest and arms up for **Locust Pose** (see page 32). Reach your palms back to your heels and press your chest forward. If your lower back feels stable, bring your legs off the floor and stretch your toes back. Take 5 deep breaths into your chest, then lower back down. Repeat 3 times.

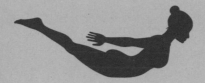

▶ For **Prone Corpse Pose** (see page 37), bend your right knee and bring it in line with your right hip. Move your arms above your head and turn your face to the right. Relax completely. Take at least 5 breaths on the right, then change sides.

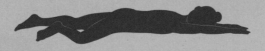

For Depression

▶ Begin by lying on your back with your knees bent and feet parallel. Bring one hand to your belly and one hand onto your lower ribs or chest. Take 5 to 10 slow, deep breaths. For each breath, exhale out completely, pause, then allow the inhalation to fill your ribs.

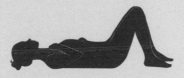

▶ Bring your elbows by your sides with your fingertips directed to the sky for **Bridge Pose** (see page 15). As you press your shoulders and upper arms into the earth, feel your collarbones widen and upper chest open. Press strongly into your feet. As you inhale, curl your tailbone up toward your knees and roll your pelvis upward. As you exhale, roll your spine back to the floor. Repeat 3 to 5 times.

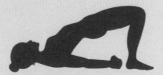

▶ Roll to one side and come onto your hands and knees. Take 5 to 10 rounds of **Cat/Cow Pose** (see page 16), focusing on timing your movement with your breathing.

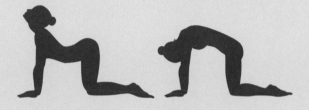

▶ Curl your toes underneath yourself and press back and up into **Downward-Facing Dog** (see page 20). As you inhale, shift forward into **Plank Pose** (see page 36). As you exhale, press back into **Downward-Facing Dog**. Repeat 3 times.

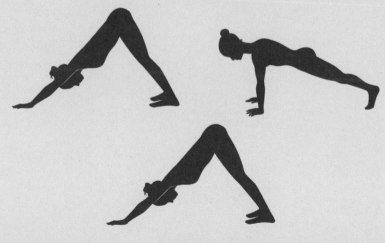

▶ The next two steps are linked into one flow. Step your right foot forward to your right thumb so that your feet are hips distance apart and parallel. Press strongly into your feet and rise up into **High-Crescent Lunge** (see page 30). Reach your arms wide to the side and then upward into a wide V position. Bring your chest and arms back. Press into your feet and sit down into your lunge, reaching your chest forward and up. Press your inner legs together and stretch through the sides of your waist as you reach your arms upward. Treat this pose like a full body yawn and stretch out in all directions. Stay for 5 deep breaths.

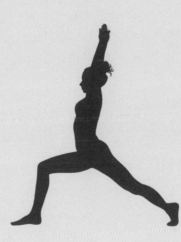

▶ Take your hands down to the floor and lower your back knee down for **Low Lunge** (see page 33). Take your left hand wide and off to the left side of your mat. Reach your right arm upward. Stretch your waist, then roll both shoulders back and downward. Turn the left side of your chest up to the sky for a twist, then scoop both shoulder blades up and into the back of your chest to bring your upper back into a backbend. If desired, you can bend your back knee and reach back toward your foot with your right hand to stretch your thigh. Take 5 deep breaths. Bring your hands back to the floor and step into **Downward-Facing Dog**. Repeat the flow on your opposite side.

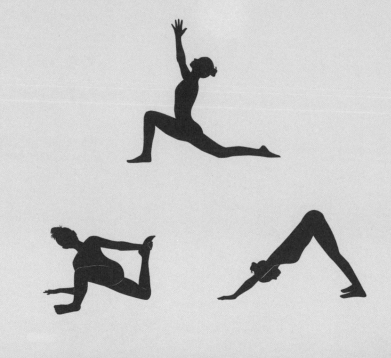

▶ Lower both knees down to the floor. Tuck your toes underneath yourself and rest on your shins to come into **Camel Pose** (see page 16). Press your inner thighs together and back as you bring your tailbone downward and engage your core. Continue through 3 rounds of **Camel Pose**, choosing the variation that works best for your body.

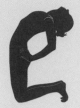

• **Variation 1:** Bring your hands together in front of your heart and lift your chest forward. Press down through your shins, continuing to press your chest forward. Lean your hips forward, still pressing your chest outward. Release your chin to your chest as you lift your sternum up. Draw your shoulders back and bring your shoulder blades up and back to expand your chest. To come out, inhale, point your feet, and sit on your heels.

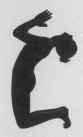

- **Variation 2:** Keeping your toes tucked underneath yourself, bring your hands onto your hips. Press down through your shins and press your chest forward. Release your chin to your chest as you lift your sternum up. Draw your shoulders back and bring your shoulder blades up and back to expand your chest. Keeping your tailbone pressed downward, reach your hands back to your heels. Press your hands into your heels and lift your sternum up to the ceiling. If your neck feels supported, you can release your head back. Take 5 deep breaths, then press into your core to lift back up onto your knees. Sit on your heels and take a few deep breaths.

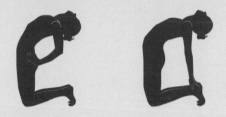

- **Variation 3:** Point your feet to deepen your backbend. Bring your hands onto your hips. Press down through your shins and press your chest forward. Release your chin to your chest as you lift your sternum up. Draw your shoulders back and bring your shoulder blades up and back to expand your chest. Press your hands into your heels and lift your sternum up to the ceiling. If your neck feels supported, you can release your head back. Press into your shins to lift your chest. Take 5 deep breaths, then press into your core to lift back up onto your knees. Sit on your heels and take a few deep breaths.

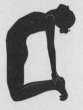

▶ Move onto all fours and come into **Cat Pose** to stretch your lower back. You can stay here, or move in **Cat/Cow Pose** to relax your spine.

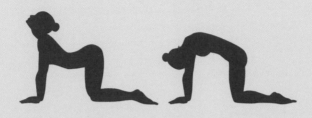

▶ Sit on your heels and come into **Hero's Pose** (see page 30) or any comfortable seated position. Bring your left hand over your heart and your right hand over your left. Feel the strength of your body and your heartbeat. As you bow your head to your heart, take a moment to thank your body for all that it does for you.

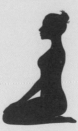

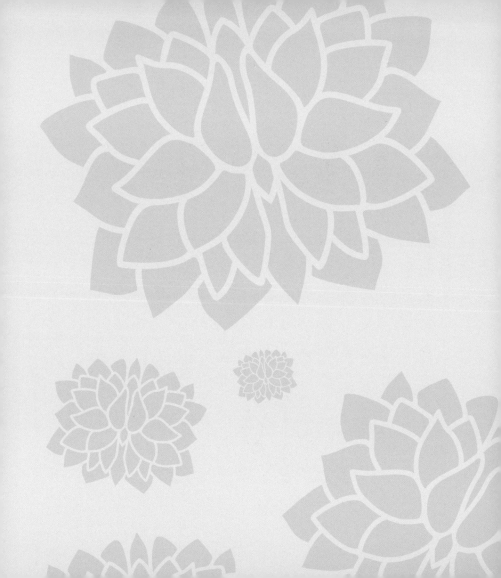

Targeted Stretches

Open Your Hip Flexors

▶ Begin in **Mountain Pose** (see page 34). Bring your hands to your heart and take 5 to 10 deep breaths to transition your attention from thinking to feeling. Open your eyes. As you inhale, reach your arms up.

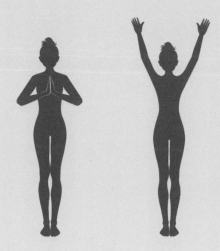

▶ As you exhale, come into **Forward Fold** (see page 25). Inhale to lift halfway up, then step your left foot back behind you so that your feet are hip distance apart. Place your hands on your front thigh and rise into **High-Crescent Lunge** (see page 30). Bend your back knee to lengthen your glutes and bring your stomach back. Keep your right hand on your front thigh and reach your left arm up and over your ear to come into a side stretch. Keeping your stomach stretched back and wide, straighten your back leg and reach through your arm. Stay for 5 to 10 breaths, stretching your left glute to open and relax the front of your hip. Bring your hands to the floor, step forward, then repeat on the opposite side.

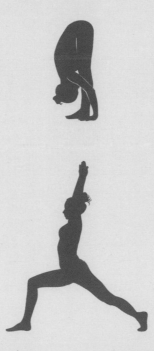

▶ From the front of your mat, step your left foot back and lower your back knee down. Place your left hand wide and off your mat. Draw your left shoulder blade outward, up, and back turning your chest upward for **Low Lunge** (see page 33). Bring your right hand upward. Stretch the sides of your throat as you press your shoulder blades back and stretch your chest into a twist/backbend combination. Press your legs toward each other and allow your pelvis to relax forward. Bring your weight above your left knee, flex your foot, and bend your knee for a thigh stretch. If desired, reach back with your right hand to hold your foot. Hold for 5 to 10 breaths, then change sides and repeat. Step back and come into **Mountain Pose**.

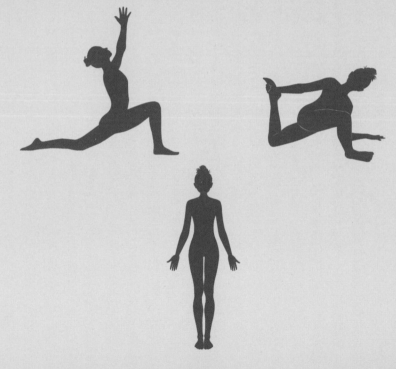

▶ As you inhale, reach your arms up. As you exhale, come into **Forward Fold** (see page 25). Inhale to lift halfway up, then step your left foot back behind you so that your feet are hip distance apart. Again, come up into **High-Crescent Lunge**, but this time, bend your back knee and press your tailbone toward the floor. Keeping your right hand on your front thigh, draw your stomach back and relax your front ribs inward. Reach your left arm upward to add a side stretch up and over to the right side. Keeping your body pressed backward, stretch your back leg out straight. Take 5 to 10 breaths, using your exhale to draw your stomach in. Inhale and reach your arms up, exhale into **Forward Fold**, then step forward to the front of your mat and repeat on the opposite side.

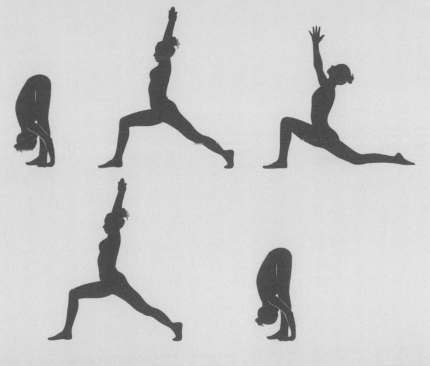

▶ Sit on your shins with your toes together and knees wide to prepare for **Saddle Pose** (see page 41). If you have difficulty bending your knees, substitute a side-lying or standing quad stretch. Place your hands behind you and lift your tailbone up toward your shins. You can walk your hands back, bring your elbows onto a support behind you, or come down onto your forearms. Keep lengthening the front of your thighs toward your knees to stretch your quadriceps. Take 10 breaths.

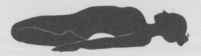

▶ Lift your chest up and bring your hands in front of you. Place your hands slightly wider than shoulder distance apart and lift up and back into **Downward-Facing Dog** (see page 20) for 3 to 5 breaths to stretch the backs of your legs. Walk forward into **Forward Fold**, then slowly rise up into **Mountain Pose**. Place your hands together in front of your heart and take a moment to appreciate your legs and all the places they take you.

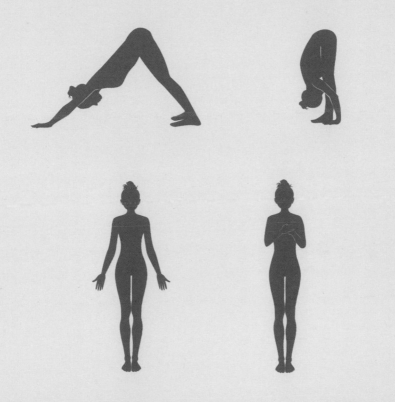

Open Your Hamstrings

This series requires a strap or a towel, some blocks, and a timer.

▶ Begin on your back in **Reclined Mountain Pose** (see page 39) with both knees bent. Take 5 long, slow breaths. Focus on the connection of your body to your mat. Draw your right knee into your chest and place a strap (or towel) around the ball of your right foot. Press your right hip into the floor and stretch your foot up to the sky for **Reclined Hand-to-Foot Pose** (see page 38). You can leave your left knee bent with your foot on the floor, or straighten your left leg and press your thigh and heel firmly down into the floor. Relax your shoulders down and allow your head to rest on the floor. Hold for two minutes, then switch sides.

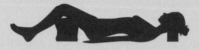

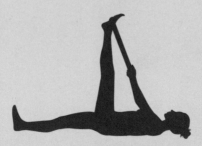

▶ Roll over onto one side and rise up onto all fours. Press firmly down into your hands, then tuck your toes underneath yourself and lift your hips up and back for **Downward-Facing Dog** (see page 20). Bend your knees and press the tops of your thighs upward. Keeping your thighs pressing upward, stretch your heels down toward the floor, and slide the balls of your feet toward the back of your mat to come into **Plank Pose** (see page 36). Stay for 10 breaths.

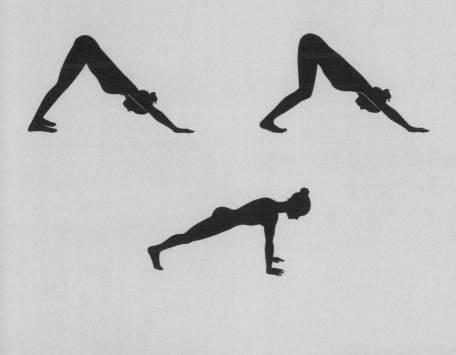

▶ Step your right foot to the front of your mat between your hands. Walk your hands to the left side of your mat and turn both of your feet to the left for **Wide-Legged Forward Fold** (see page 52). Ensure that your feet are parallel to each other and bring your weight forward into the balls of your feet. Soften the backs of your knees as you lift through the backs of your legs. Release your upper body and head toward the floor. Stay for 10 breaths.

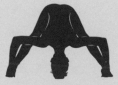

▶ Walk your feet toward each other until they are parallel and hip distance apart to come into **Forward Fold** (see page 25). Hold on to your opposite elbows and bend your knees so that your upper body can release toward the floor. Take 5 breaths, then switch the crossing of your arms. After 5 more breaths, release your arms to the floor and slowly roll up to stand. Stand in **Mountain Pose** (see page 34), bring your hands to your heart, and take 2 to 3 centering breaths through your whole body.

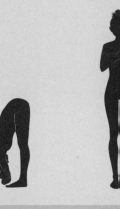

OPEN YOUR SHOULDERS

This series requires a strap or a towel at the front of your mat.

▶ Stand in **Mountain Pose** (see page 34) and take 3 to 5 deep, clearing breaths to make a transition from thinking to feeling. To begin **Sun Salutation A** (see page 45), inhale and reach your arms up into **Upward Salute** (see page 49). Exhale into **Forward Fold** (see page 25), then inhale into **Halfway Lift** (see page 29). As you exhale, step back into **Plank Pose** (see page 36) and lower all the way to the earth. You can keep your knees straight if you wish. Inhale into a backbend like **Baby Cobra** (see page 15) or **Upward-Facing Dog** (see page 50), then exhale into **Downward-Facing Dog** (see page 20). Take 5 breaths.

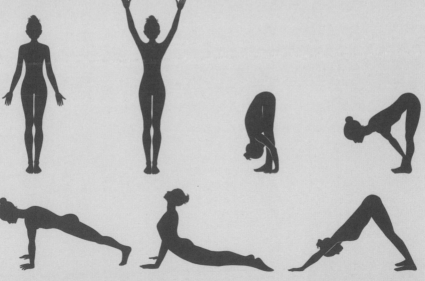

▶ Inhale, step to the front of your mat, and come into **Halfway Lift**. Exhale into **Forward Fold**. Inhale, stand up, and reach your arms up into **Upward Salute**. Exhale and bring your hands to your sides. Repeat 2 to 4 times, focusing on the movement of your arms and breath. On your last round, stay in **Downward-Facing Dog**.

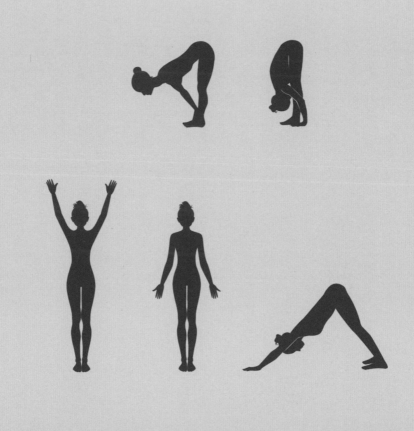

▶ From **Downward-Facing Dog**, step your right foot to your right hand so that your feet are hip distance apart and parallel. Using the strap, rise up into **High-Crescent Lunge** (see page 30). Bend your back knee slightly so that you can bring your tailbone downward. Hold the strap behind your back with your palms facing forward and your hands about shoulder distance apart. Relax your front ribs in slightly and draw your shoulders back. Keeping your core tensed, press your shoulders outward and stretch your arms back behind you. Continue to pull the strap apart as you reach your chest forward and up. Take 5 to 10 deep breaths into your upper chest to stretch your shoulders. Release the strap, bring your hands to the floor, and step forward. Then, step your right foot back and repeat on the second side. When finished, step back into **Downward-Facing Dog**.

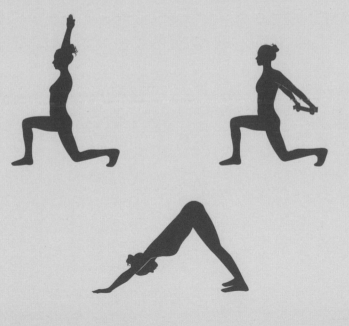

▶ From **Downward-Facing Dog**, step your right foot to your right hand so that your feet are hip distance apart and parallel. Using the strap, rise up into **High-Crescent Lunge**. Bend your back knee slightly to stretch your tailbone downward. Reach your left arm up to the sky. Use your right hand to pull your left arm forward, then bend your left elbow and bring your hands to the middle of your back for a triceps stretch. If you are more flexible in your shoulders, you can bring your hand to your left shoulder blade. Use your right hand to bring your left arm in. Press your left shoulder back and out as you stretch through your left elbow. Take 5 breaths. Release your hands to the floor, step back into **Downward-Facing Dog**, then repeat on the opposite side.

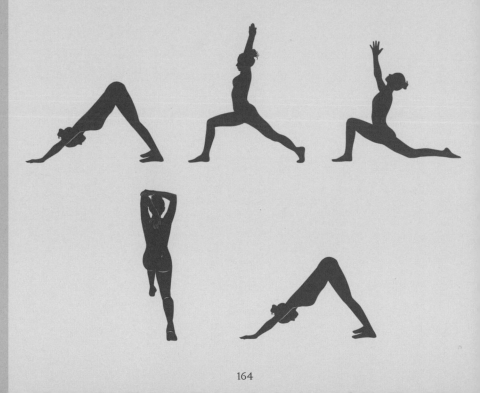

▶ Step to the front of your mat into a **Forward Fold** and interlace your hands behind your back. If you need more space for your shoulders in the stretch, hold the strap between your hands. Bend your elbows, lift your shoulders up, and stretch your hands upward. Focus on keeping your shoulders lifted. Your elbows can remain bent with your palms apart. If you have more shoulder flexibility, you may eventually straighten your elbows and press your palms together. Take 5 deep breaths. Roll up slowly into a standing position.

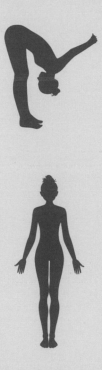

▶ Inhale and reach your arms out wide. As you exhale, cross your arms in front of you with your right arm under your left and hold onto your opposite shoulders. Stay here, press the backs of your forearms into each other, or wrap your forearms and press your palms together like in **Eagle Pose** (see page 20). You can also bend your knees, rotate your right thigh inward, and lift and cross your right thigh over your left, pressing your shins together. Lift your forearms up and press them slightly forward to stretch your shoulders. Stay for 5 breaths, then unwind your arms and legs and switch sides.

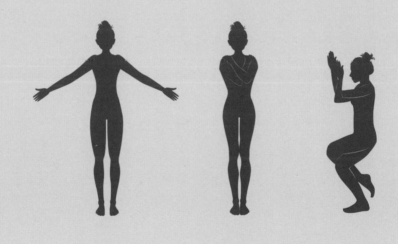

▶ Stand in **Mountain Pose** with your feet hip distance apart. Hold the strap slightly wider than shoulder width apart. For this exercise, you can allow your hands to slide apart as far as you need on the strap, but keep your arms straight. As you inhale, lift your arms overhead. As you exhale, make a giant circle through your shoulders to bring your arms back behind you. Then, inhale and pull the strap apart as you lift your arms back upward. Exhale and bring your hands to your sides. Repeat 4 times. Stand in **Mountain Pose** and take 3 to 5 breaths, appreciating the openness in your chest, ribs, and shoulders.

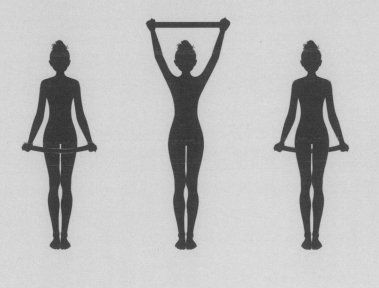

Open Your Outer Hips

▶ Begin in **Easy Seat** (see page 21) with your shins crossed and your feet under your knees. You may wish to sit on a block, book, or pillow to lift your hips. Use your hands to press your glutes wide and slightly back in order to sit upright on your tailbone. Bring your hands to your heart and take a few centering breaths.

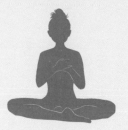

▶ Bring your fingertips behind you. Inhale and lift your chest. As you exhale, come into a **Forward Fold** (see page 25) over your cross-legged seat. If you can easily lengthen your chest forward, bring your hands in front of you and allow your spine to relax forward and down. Let your head relax and feel the stretch through your outer hips. Take 10 deep breaths. On your next inhale, rise up, change which shin is in front, and repeat on the opposite side.

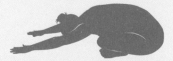

▶ Begin on all fours for 5 rounds of **Cat/Cow Pose** (see page 16). Curl your toes underneath yourself and press backward into **Downward-Facing Dog** (see page 20). Hold for 3 to 5 breaths.

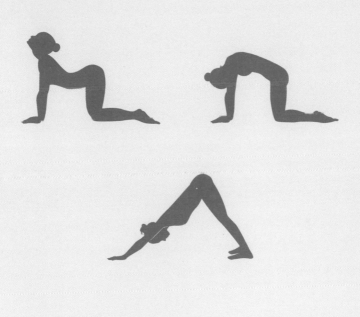

▶ Step your right foot between your hands, turn your left heel down parallel to the back of your mat, and rotate your arms upward into **Warrior 2** (see page 51). As you press your left thigh straight, press your right hip down toward the floor and press your right knee outward to stretch your right glute. Hold for 10 breaths. Rotate your hands down to the floor and step back into **Downward-Facing Dog**. Repeat on the opposite side.

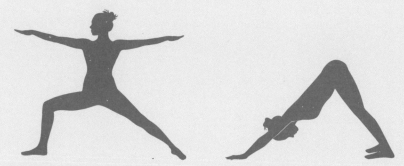

▶ Sit on the floor and bring your right shin parallel to the front edge of your mat. Bring your back shin parallel to the left long edge of your mat, keeping each leg at a right angle and inhale. As you exhale, fold forward over your front leg for a variation of **Pigeon Pose** (see page 36). Keep your right hip pressed on the floor. You can adjust the angle of your front shin by moving your knee wider to the right or left, as well as adjust the angle of your body. If you can keep your right hip down, you may also slide your left foot back toward the back of your mat to increase the stretch on the front outer hip. If you feel any knee pain or pressure, discontinue this pose and opt for **Eye of the Needle Pose** (see page 24) instead. Hold for 20 breaths, then change sides.

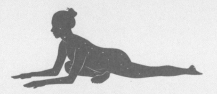

▶ As you come out, sit on your left hip. Move your left knee slightly toward the center of your mat so that your knee is now in line with your pubic bone rather than your outer hip. Swing your right leg forward and bring it up and over your left leg, stacking your knees for **Cow Face Pose** (see page 19). Your hips should remain grounded and your ankles should be near your hips. It is okay if your knees are not completely crossed, so long as your knees feel comfortable. If you are having trouble, sit on a block or attempt the pose in a reclined position. Inhale to stretch upward. Exhale and fold forward and hold for 20 breaths. Straighten your legs, then repeat on the opposite side.

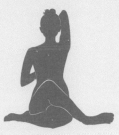

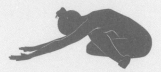

Mobilize Your Spine

▶ Begin in **Extended Child's Pose** (see page 23) with your knees wide, your hips on your heels, and your upper body relaxed toward the earth. Take 5 deep breaths to center yourself. Keeping your hips on your heels, walk your hands toward the right side of your mat for a lateral spinal stretch. Take 5 deep breaths, then move to the opposite side.

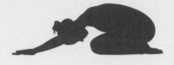

▶ Inhale, rise up onto all fours, and come into **Cat/Cow Pose** (see page 16), feeling the stretch through your whole body After a few rounds, explore different movements in the pose, such as rolling through your shoulders and shifting your hips from side to side.

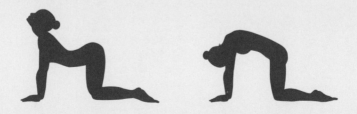

▶ Curl your toes underneath yourself and lift your hips up and back into **Downward-Facing Dog** (see page 20). Press firmly into your hands, bend your knees, and stretch your hips upward. Push your thighs up and back, simultaneously reaching your chest outward toward your thumbs to lengthen your stomach. Hold for 10 breaths.

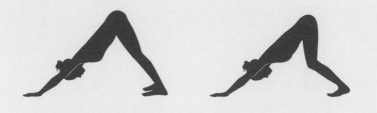

▶ Inhale and come into **Plank Pose** (see page 36). As you exhale, lower down into **Locust Pose** (see page 32). Stretch both your legs back hip distance apart and press the tops of your feet down. Roll your inner thighs upward and stretch your tailbone back to your heels. Reach your arms behind you and interlace your hands. Feel free to keep your hands free if interlacing them causes strain on your shoulders. Lift your shoulders upward, pressing them outward as you lift. As you inhale, lift up through your chest and legs, draw your hands toward your heels, and relax your chest forward. Take 3 breaths, focusing on stretching your back with every inhale. Lower down, then repeat 2 times.

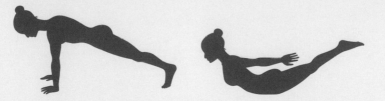

▶ Prop yourself up on your forearms so that your elbows are under your shoulders for **Sphinx Pose** (see page 43). If you have any lower back discomfort, move your elbows further forward so that your lower ribs can stay on your mat. Stretch your tailbone back. Press your forearms down and pull your palms back to open your chest and widen your collarbones. For a deeper backbend, lift your elbows and continue to move your chest forward and up. Stay for 5 breaths, drawing your upper back forward and opening your chest as you inhale. Lower your body to the earth and look to one side.

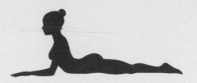

▶ When you are ready, press up and back into **Downward-Facing Dog**. Then, step your right foot between your hands. Lower your back knee down. Place your hands at the center of your chest. Inhale to lengthen your chest, and as you exhale, twist to the right to place your left elbow outside your knee for **Revolved Lunge** (see page 40). You may leave your back knee down, or lift it for stability. Remain for 5 breaths, focusing on your spinal stretch. Then, lower your hands, move back into **Downward-Facing Dog**, and change sides.

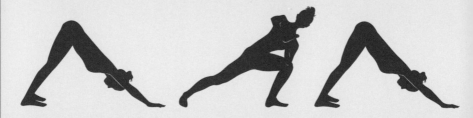

▶ Step forward to the front of your mat. Bend your knees and hinge forward into **Forward Fold** (see page 25), allowing your upper body to relax fully. Remain for 5 breaths, then take 3 slow breaths to roll up through your spine to a standing position. Stand in **Mountain Pose** (see page 34), bring your hands to your heart, and take 5 slow, deep breaths.

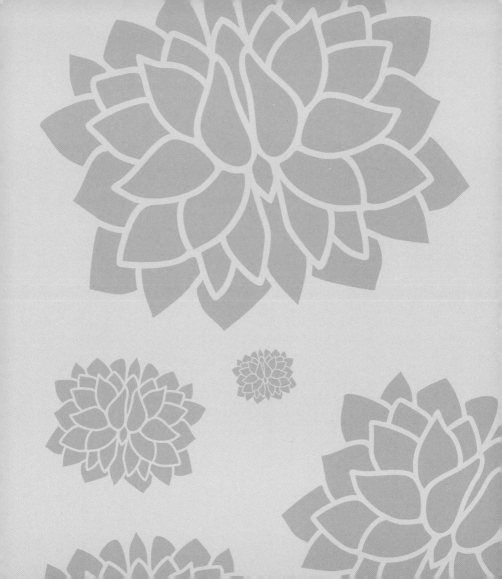

Desk Medicine

Seated Neck Therapy

▶ Sitting tall on the edge of your chair, roll your shoulders up, back, and down about 5 times. Then, repeat in the opposite direction. Keeping your chest lifted, lower your right ear to your right shoulder to stretch the side of your neck. Draw your chin slightly down to your right shoulder to stretch different parts of your neck, and pause when you find a good spot. If desired, reach your left fingertips wide to the left to increase the stretch, or add gentle pressure to your neck by placing your right hand on your head. Take 5 to 10 deep breaths. Repeat on your right side.

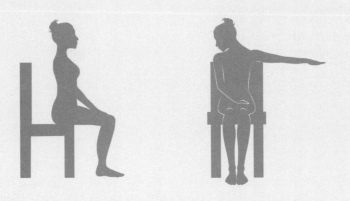

▶ Keep your chest lifted and broad as you release your chin to your chest to stretch the back of your neck. Either let the weight of your head do the work for you, or deepen your stretch by gently interlacing your hands on the back of your head. Keeping your chest open, slowly draw your chin from the center of your chest in a semi-circle to each shoulder to stretch the back of your neck. Take about 20 breaths.

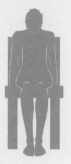

▶ Place one hand on your heart and the other hand over that hand. Lift your chin slightly up and to the right. Jut your lower jaw forward to stretch your scalenes at the front and sides of the throat. The back of your neck in this pose should stay long and supported. Take 10 breaths on each side. When you change sides, change which hand in on top. Sit and take 5 slow, deep breaths.

Leg Wake Up

▶ Stand in **Mountain Pose** (see page 34) with your feet hip distance apart and parallel. Take 3 deep inhales and exhales. Bend your knees, bring your weight into your heels, and reach your arms forward and up into **Chair Pose** (see page 17). As you send your hips back and down, stretch your arms forward and up to help lengthen your spine. Deepen the stretch by bending your knees and arms and straightening them. Do this 10 times, working a little bit deeper into your chair each time.

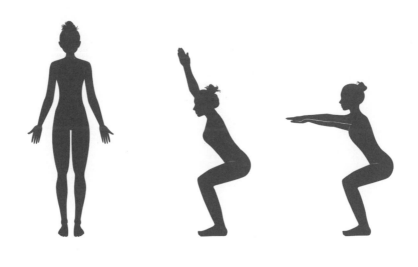

▶ Exhale into **Forward Fold** (see page 25) over your legs. Release your upper body toward the floor and turn your head side to side to release any tension in your neck. Stretch your face into a yawn to release any jaw and facial tension, being sure to exhale through your mouth.

▶ Bring your hands to the floor and step your left foot far back. Place your feet hip distance apart and parallel. Bring your hands onto your front thigh and inhale to rise up into a **High-Crescent Lunge** (see page 30). Reach your arms upward. Bend your back knee, hover it off the floor, and inhale. As you exhale, press your hands down toward the floor. Press your legs together and straighten them. Inhale, bend your back knee, and reach your arms up. Repeat this moving **High-Crescent Lunge** 5 times. Bring your hands to the floor for balance, step forward, then step your right foot back and repeat on the opposite side.

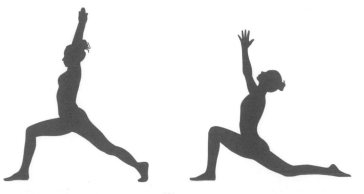

▶ Come back into **Chair Pose** at the front of your mat with your hands pressed together in front of your heart. Inhale to stretch your spine. As you exhale, twist to the right, bringing your left elbow across your right knee into **Revolved Chair Pose** (see page 40). Bring your hips lower and lift and open your chest. Keep your knees even. Press your elbow and knee together and lift your left foot off the floor to practice your balance. Stay for 5 breaths. Inhale to untwist into a **Forward Fold**, then repeat on the opposite side.

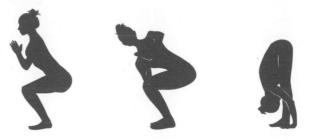

▶ Slowly roll up through your spine into **Mountain Pose**. Bend your knees slightly so that you can feel the weight of your body settle onto your legs. Take 3 deep breaths and appreciate the time you took to practice.

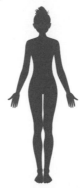

Seated Spinal Stretches

▶ Begin seated at the edge of your chair with your feet flat on the floor. Roll your shoulders up, back, and down a few times and take 3 deep breaths.

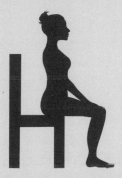

▶ Bringing your hands on either the edge or your chair or your arm rests, take 5 to 10 rounds of seated **Cat/Cow Pose** (see page 16), focusing on arching and rounding your spine.

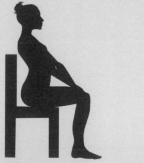
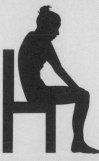

▶ Interlace your hands and press your palms forward, stretching your shoulders outward. Press your hips down and your palms up to the sky for **Upward Salute** (see page 49). Bring your bottom ribs in as you draw your arms back and straight. Take 5 breaths, then lower your hands, interlace your fingers the opposite way, and repeat on your opposite side.

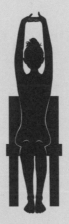

▶ Press your legs together. Inhale, then as you exhale, kick your right heel forward. Stretch your heel fully in front of you, sit tall, and hold for 5 full, deep breaths. Repeat on your opposite side.

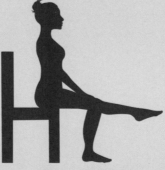

▶ Inhale and reach your arms up. As you exhale, twist to the right. Depending on your chair, you can either hold on to the back of your chair, or your arm rest. As you inhale, lengthen your back. As you exhale, twist. Stay for 5 breaths, deepening the stretch with each breath. Inhale back to center and reach your arms up. Repeat on the left side. Return to a tall, seated position and take 3 deep breaths, appreciating the openness of your body.

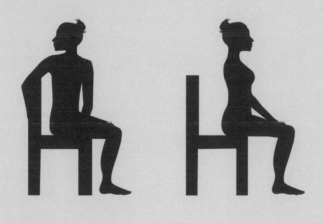

Anti-Desk Practice

▶ Stand in **Mountain Pose** (see page 34) with your feet hip distance apart and parallel and take 3 deep, clearing breaths. Begin **Interrupted Breathing Exercise** (see page 31). As you inhale, reach your arms wide and up, press your palms together, and gaze up to your fingers. As you exhale, slowly drag your pressed palms down through the center of your body. At about your stomach, interlace your hands and press your palms toward the floor. Follow your hands with your gaze. Repeat 5 to 10 times.

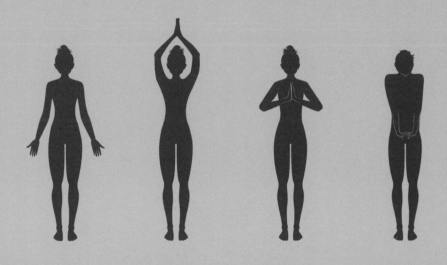

▶ Reach your arms wide and upward to come into **Standing Side Bend** (see page 44). Turn your right palm up and hold onto your right wrist with your left hand. Shifting your hips to the right, take a giant side stretch over to the left. To deepen your stretch, experiment with taking your left foot off the floor. Take 5 breaths, then repeat on the opposite side.

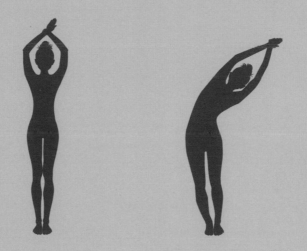

▶ Interlace your hands behind your back and roll your shoulders up, back, and down. As you reach your palms back behind you, shift your weight forward into your toes, and lift your chest forward and up into **Standing Backbend** (see page 43). Lower your chin slightly to keep the back of your neck long, relax your jaw, and lift your shoulder blades up and back. Take 5 deep breaths into your upper chest. Change the interlace of your fingers and repeat.

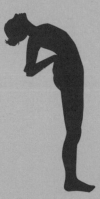

▶ Bring your feet and legs together, bend your knees, and sit into **Chair Pose** (see page 17). Bring your weight back into you heels as you stretch your arms forward and up. Drop your shoulders outward as you stretch your arms forward and extend through your fingertips. Stand up into **Mountain Pose**, with your palms facing outward. Take 5 deep breaths and appreciate the openness of your body.

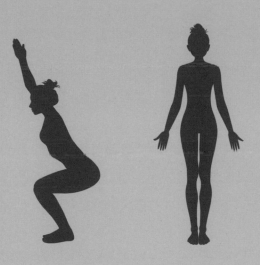

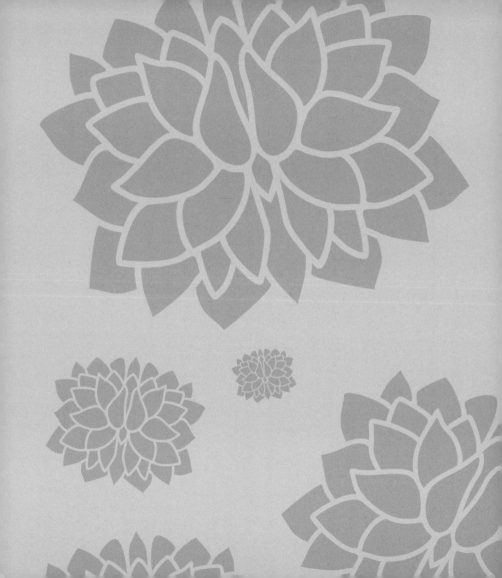

One Minute Miracles

Quick Wake Up

▶ To begin **Skull-Shining Breath** (see page 42), sit either on the floor, on a block, or on the edge of a chair. Lift tall through your spine and reach your arms overhead in a wide V position. Take a deep inhale, then exhale out fully. Inhale halfway, then begin a series of short, sharp exhales through your nose at a rate of about 1 to 2 per second. Allow your inhales to drop in naturally and keep your chest lifted and open. Exhale 25 times. Take a few natural breaths in and out.

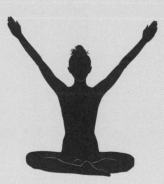

► The next two poses are linked. To begin **Half Sun Salutation** (see page 28), inhale to lift your arms up into **Upward Salute** (see page 49), then exhale into **Forward Fold** (see page 25). Inhale into **Halfway Lift** (see page 29), then exhale and step your left foot back for a long lunge with your feet hip distance apart and parallel. If desired, lower your back knee. Bring your hands together in front of your heart. Inhale, lengthen your upper body, and exhale and twist to the right for **Revolved Side Angle Pose** (see page 41), bringing your left elbow outside your right knee. Take 3 breaths.

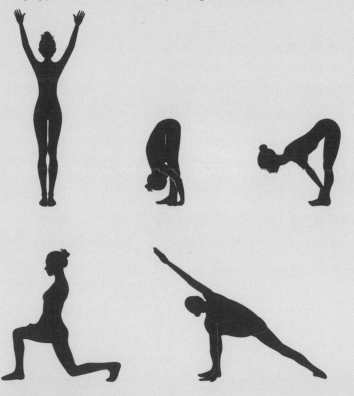

▶ Inhale to untwist and place your hands on either side of your front foot. If desired, lower your back knee. Pull your hips back, straighten your front leg, and fold forward into a variation of **Pyramid Pose** (see page 37). Take 3 breaths. If desired, flex your front foot and pull your toes upward. Bend your front knee and step forward, then repeat on your opposite side.

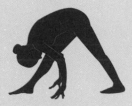

▶ Stand in **Mountain Pose** (see page 34) and take 3 deep breaths.

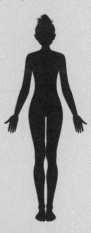

Quick Spinal Decompression

▶ Begin on all fours, then curl your toes underneath yourself and lift your hips up and back into **Downward-Facing Dog** (see page 20). Bend your knees and draw the tops of your thighs up and back. Keeping your hips lifted, press strongly into your inner hands and reach your chest toward your thumbs to lengthen both sides of your waist. If desired, bend a knee or press back into your heel to stretch your calves. You can also shift both heels from right to left and back again to stretch your waist.

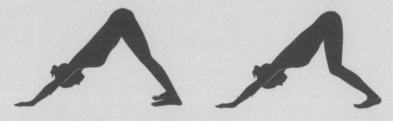

▶ Walk your hands back to your feet, bend your knees, and allow your upper body to hang over your lower body into **Forward Fold** (see page 25). Turn your head side to side to release your neck. Sway side to side to release tension in your spine, if desired, bending your knees several time to help relax your whole body.

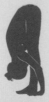

▶ Keeping your head and arms completely relaxed, slowly roll up through your spine over the course of 4 to 5 breaths, shifting your weight to your feet. If you become lightheaded, **Forward Fold** once more and move slower until your body can equalize. Once you come into **Mountain Pose** (see page 34), roll your shoulders up, back, and down several times to relax your neck.

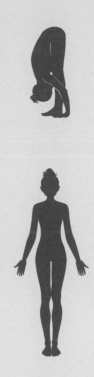

▶ Place your hands on a wall shoulder distance apart with your hands at at hip height and step back into an L-shaped pose to come into a variation of **Warrior 3** (see page 51). Press into your hands, bend your knees slightly, and pull your hips back toward the center of the room to lengthen your spine. Keeping your spine straight, hug your feet and legs together, and begin to straighten your legs. Keeping your arms straight and your pelvis square to the floor, reach your right leg back toward the center of the room for 5 breaths. Lower your right leg, then lift your left leg for 5 breaths. Keep your arms and legs straight. Lower your leg, stand up, take a few deep breaths, and appreciate your newly relaxed body.

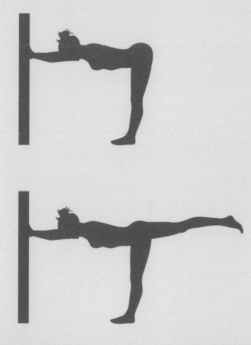

INSTANT DE-STRESS

▶ To begin **Half Sun Salutation** (see page 28), inhale and reach your arms upward for **Upward Salute** (see page 49). Exhale, bend your knees slightly, and **Forward Fold** (see page 25). Inhale and come into **Halfway Lift** (see page 29). Exhale back into **Forward Fold**. Inhale and reach your arms upward. Exhale and move your hands to your sides. Repeat 3 times, focusing on connecting your movement to your breathing.

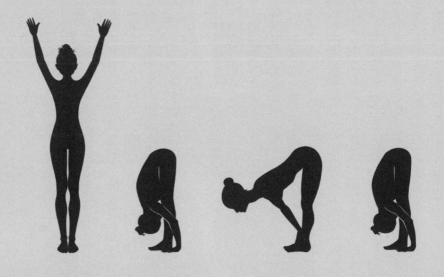

▶ Come up into **Mountain Pose** (see page 34) with your hands over your heart. Feel your heartbeat. Inhale for a count of 4, then exhale for a count of 6. Pause between each breath. Repeat 5 times.

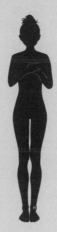

ONE MINUTE UNWIND

▶ To begin **Legs-Up-the-Wall Pose** (see page 32), lay on your back with your legs against the wall. If you have tight hamstrings, position your pelvis 1 to 2 feet from the wall. You can also use a strap or tie a scarf around your thighs so that your legs can completely relax.

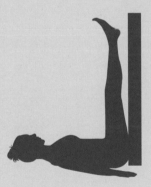

▶ Place one hand on your belly and one hand on your lower ribs. Take a full, complete breath in and out to prepare for a breathing exercise. To begin, take a modest inhale into your belly. Pause. Take a modest inhale into your lower ribs. Pause. Take a final inhale into your upper chest. Pause. Exhale all the way out. Repeat this for 6 rounds, then return to your natural breathing. When you're ready, slowly roll over onto one side and sit up.

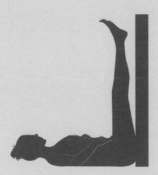

HAPPY HEART OPENER

▶ Start in **Mountain Pose** (see page 34) and take 3 deep breaths. Reach your arms up overhead, turn your right palm upward, and hold onto your right wrist with your left hand. Relax your shoulders and press your tailbone downward. Lean into your right foot and curve your left side up and over to the left into an arch, bending at the waist. To deepen this side stretch, lift your left foot. Hold for 3 breaths, then change sides.

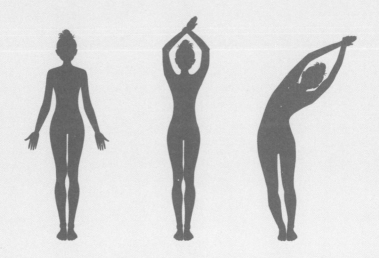

▶ Inhale and reach your arms up, then exhale into **Forward Fold** (see page 25). Inhale to come into **Halfway Lift** (see page 29), then exhale and step your left foot back. Rise up into **High-Crescent Lunge** (see page 30). Interlace your hands behind your head and point your elbows forward to relax your shoulders outward.

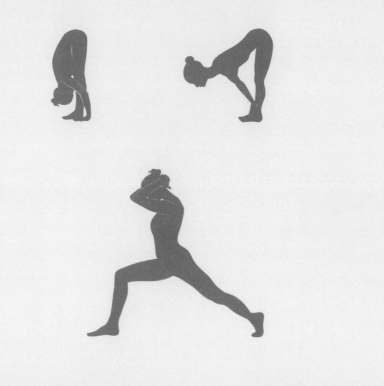

▶ Balance back onto your legs, keeping your weight centered over them. Press your chest back, tense your left glute, and straighten your back leg. Press your head into your hands and reach your chest forward and up. Take a deep breath. Lean into the ball of your back foot and push your front heel down to lift your stomach up. Tense your core as you exhale, then inhale to reach your arms straight upward. On your next exhale, press into your feet and bring your hands to the floor. Step forward, come into **Forward Fold**, and take 3 breaths. Step your right foot back and repeat **High-Crescent Lunge** on the opposite side.

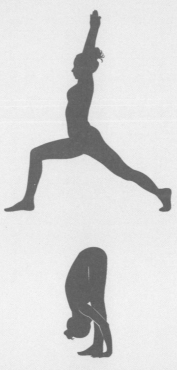

▶ As you step to the front of your mat, inhale and come into **Halfway Lift**. Bring your hands to your hips, then inhale and stand up. Place your hands on your heart in **Mountain Pose** and hold as long as feels nourishing.

ABOUT THE AUTHOR

A yoga teacher, mentor, and educator, Rachel Scott helps teachers and studios around the world to create teacher trainings and continuing education programs. Her extensive knowledge and experience include earning two masters degrees, authoring three books, and leading over 4,000 hours of teacher training. As a writer and speaker, she continually wrestles with the juicy bits of life: relationships, authenticity, and discovering meaning in this crazy, wonderful world. She holds an E-RYT 500, YACEP, BA, MFA, and MSci and is a wicked coffee drinker. Find Rachel and enjoy her tips, classes, and musings at www.rachelyoga.com.

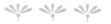

About Cider Mill Press
Book Publishers

Good ideas ripen with time. From seed to harvest, Cider Mill Press brings fine reading, information, and entertainment together between the covers of its creatively crafted books. Our Cider Mill bears fruit twice a year, publishing a new crop of titles each spring and fall.

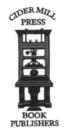

"Where Good Books Are Ready for Press"

Visit us on the web at
www.cidermillpress.com
or write to us at
PO Box 454
12 Spring St.
Kennebunkport, Maine 04046